PRAISE FOR

HEALTHY BODY CONNECTION

Kudos to Lee Bomzer for penning a remarkable and detailed book. Read it and you will be both informed and inspired to begin the journey to optimize your health and wellbeing, and living a life well-grounded and suffused with joy.

Sanjiv Chopra MD.

Bestselling author and sought after inspirational speaker.

An adventurous exploration into Lee´s world and views on keeping a healthy relationship with our foods, the importance of good sleep and exercise, the avoidance of stress to hinder weight gain, inflammation and chronic illnesses. *Healthy Body Connection* is full of practical information combined with references to the latest research within the field. Wondering how to live your life in harmony, with balance between your inner and outer life? Read this book! – it gave me a really good gut feeling!

-Gunnar Rafn Jónsson, MD

Healthy Body Connection is a compelling read, a book that empowers people to take control of their futures by understanding that true health is a state of complete physical, mental, and social well-being.

Dr. Kailash Chand OBE

Honorary Vice President of the British Medical Association,
and ex-chair of Tameside and Glossop NHS

Healthy Body Connection is part instruction manual, and part informational guide. It's easy to follow, interesting, engaging, and well-researched. Lee has developed a simple plan for you to change your life – and keep the changes going

Rina Meyer, MD

Assistant Professor of Clinical Pediatrics

Division of Pediatric Hematology and Oncology,

Stony Brook University School of Medicine

In her well-referenced book, *Healthy Body Connection,* Lee Bomzer skillfully weaves in up-to-date science, resulting in a powerful, yet accessible plan to help you create a happy, healthy body for life.

Vincent Pedre M.D.

Author of the best-selling book, *Happy Gut*

HEALTHY BODY CONNECTION

Unlocking Your Body's Natural Connection

to

Sustainable Weight Loss and Optimal Health

Lee Bomzer

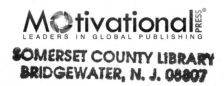

Published by Motivational Press, Inc.
1777 Aurora Road
Melbourne, Florida, 32935
www.MotivationalPress.com

Manufactured in the United States of America.

ISBN: 978-1-62865-492-9

NOTICE

All matters regarding your health should be discussed with your doctor.

Not all of the information, statements, advice, opinions, or suggestions set forth in the material referenced or contained in this book have been evaluated by the FDA, and should not be relied upon to diagnose, treat, cure, or prevent any condition or disease.

This book represents the research and ideas of the author concerning diet, nutrition, exercise, and lifestyle. This book is written as a source of information only, and not as a medical manual. The information presented in the following pages is designed to help you make informed decisions about your health. The recommendations in this book are not intended to replace or conflict with the advice given to you by your physician or other health professionals. If you suspect that you have a medical problem, we urge you to seek competent medical care.

Consult your physician before adopting the suggestions in this book. Following these dietary suggestions may impact the effect of certain types of medication. Any changes in dosage should be made only in cooperation with your prescribing physician. Your doctor should always be consulted before beginning any new diet, exercise, therapeutic, or other health program.

Additionally, the information in this book is meant to supplement, not replace, proper exercise training. All forms of exercise pose some inherent risks. The author, editors, and publisher, advise readers to take full responsibility for their safety and know their limits. Before practicing the exercises in this book, be sure that your equipment is well-maintained, and do not take risks beyond your level of experience, aptitude, training, and fitness. The exercise and dietary programs in this book are not intended as a substitute for any exercise routine or dietary regime that may have been prescribed by your doctor. Again, as with all exercise and dietary programs, you should get your doctor's approval before beginning

The author accepts no responsibility for the use of any information or material contained in this book. The author and the publisher expressly disclaim responsibility for any adverse effects arising from the use or application of the information contained herein, by any person.

Mention of specific companies, organizations, or authorities in this book does not imply endorsement by the author or publisher, nor does mention of specific companies, organizations, or authorities imply that they endorse this book, its author, or the publisher.

All efforts have been made to ensure the accuracy of the information contained in this book as of the date published, neither the publisher nor the author assumes any responsibility for errors, or for changes that occur after publication.

Further, the author and publisher do not have any control over and do not assume any responsibility for third party websites or their content. Any internet addresses and telephone numbers given in this book were accurate at the time it went to press.

To my BFF, Selma Bomzer, who passed on before this book was finished, and to my beautiful sister, Robin Lori.

Words cannot express my gratitude for having had you in my life.

By example, you have each shown me what it is to live a full life, and a life of merit.

Neither one of you ever asked for anything in return for all that you gave.

Individually, you have inspired me, and taught me the true meanings of love, grace, strength, beauty, and generosity.

I see the world differently for having known you both, and I am grateful.

Your love, your smiles, and your laughter, will be missed, but never forgotten.

I will remember you and keep you in my heart, always.

I am a thousand winds that blow,
I am the diamond glints on snow,
I am the sun on ripened grain,
I am the gentle autumn rain.
When you awaken in the morning's hush,
I am the swift uplifting rush
Of quiet birds in circled flight.
I am the soft stars that shine at night.

- Excerpt from (Do not stand at my grave and weep), a poem by Mary Elizabeth Frye, 1932

CONTENTS

FOREWORD

I HAVE TO ADMIT IT — as an oncologist, I am always a little skeptical of books about health and healthy living. I am always on the lookout for inaccurate information or pseudoscience. But, you won't find any of that in this book. *Healthy Body Connection* is a refreshing change from your run-of-the-mill lifestyle book — Lee Bomzer takes her role as your health coach seriously. This book is different because Lee isn't just writing about her own experience (although it beautifully colors the work) and she isn't just quoting a few things she read on the internet. *Healthy Body Connection* is rigorously researched, using primary sources from the medical literature. It's responsibly written; it's reliable and, most importantly, it's both interesting and do-able. *Healthy Body Connection* will make you rethink what you know about eating well, exercise, and your relationship with yourself.

When you're trying to change your life, you may feel overwhelmed. Every website, TV show, book, magazine, and podcast has advice for you — some of it contradicting, some of it confusing. *Healthy Body Connection* simplifies the path for you. In this book, Lee merges her own story with interesting tidbits of research and biology, along with a clear and simple plan to become healthier in a sustainable way. This is not a "diet book." It's a recipe for a healthier life, a plan to becoming your best you! Everything you need to change your life is right here at your fingertips — what foods work best and why, how to move your body, information on mindfulness, and some delicious new recipes. (I think I am finally excited about eating turkey burgers!)

We are so fortunate to live in a time where medicine has never been more advanced, but yet, we continue to see chronic illnesses ruining the lives of ourselves and those we love. And while modern medicine has many wonderful answers that save lives, it doesn't have them all. As a physician, I understand the value of merging our medical knowledge with common sense – good nutrition, regular movement, balance, and mindfulness. It's not "this or that" - it's "this AND that" that will make our society healthier again. Not every health coach understands that – Lee does. Lee's understanding of this principle is at the core of *Healthy Body Connection* – simply put, it's why this book works.

Healthy Body Connection is part instruction manual, and part informational guide. It's easy to follow, interesting, engaging, and well-researched. Lee has developed a simple plan for you to change your life – and keep the changes going. I hope you enjoy it and learn as much from it as I did!

Rina Meyer, MD
Assistant Professor of Clinical Pediatrics
Division of Pediatric Hematology and Oncology
Stony Brook University School of Medicine

PROLOGUE

COMFORTABLE SUFFERING

"Our genes are not our destiny. Our genes load the gun; but it's our environment that pulls the trigger."

- Dr. Rangan Chatterjee

WHEN WE ARE SUFFERING from a non-communicable or chronic disease, modern medicine seeks to give us comfort. The result is that we comfortably suffer.

I wrote this book because it doesn't have to be this way. I've learned that we each have the potential to have a more fulfilling, happier, and healthier life. We can unlock our body's natural connection to sustainable weight loss and optimal health, and our lives on purpose. We don't have to accept a life of comfortable suffering. Through intentional changes in lifestyle and nutrition, we have the power to positively influence our genes, prevent, and reverse chronic disease, increase our life spans, and improve the overall quality of our lives.

If you use the strategies that I offer within the pages of this book, you will likely lose a substantial amount of excess weight, but weight loss of itself is not the goal. The number one objective of this plan, is to keep the possibility of comfortable suffering, out your life.

So, what I offer you is not a diet book, but an invitation to add more years to your life, and more life to your years. Not through a quick fix, or a temporary resolution, but through a reasonable, and lasting, personalized nutritional & lifestyle plan.

INTRODUCTION

RECENTLY A LOT OF NEW information has been circulating in the news, on talk shows, and in social media about how we can achieve our best health, avoid chronic disease, lose weight, and avoid the illnesses that we may be genetically predisposed to. This information has been disseminated to us by many renowned researchers, doctors, and experts in the field of medicine. They tell us that we can accomplish all of this by following specific dietary and lifestyle recommendations. Many of them have written books and produced video symposiums for public consumption. Additionally, there have been, and continue to be, many recent conferences where scientists, researchers, clinicians, health care providers, and doctors, get together to share the latest on new technology, scientific breakthroughs, studies, and newly acquired knowledge, with one another.

Amazingly, with so many great minds at work there are a myriad of things that they all can agree on. As a matter, of course however, there are also a bunch of things that they disagree on. For example, some will counsel you to eat meat, while others advise against consuming meat. Some advocate enjoying full fat dairy, while others have taken dairy off the table for good, and still others recommend consuming dairy only if it's low fat. The same is true of beans, certain fruits, fats, oils, and even exercise! So how is a reasonable person to know what to do? Whose advice should you listen to? Which plan is going to serve you best? How can you achieve the promised ultimate health, wellbeing, and ideal body weight?

As a person, whose deepest desire is to help myself, my loved ones, and as many others as I can, to live a healthy life free of unnecessary illness and suffering, and as a health coach, who wants to give her clients the very best care and information, those are the questions I needed to answer.

I decided that the best way to answer those questions for myself, would be to gather as much information on the subject as I could. One good way to start was by getting input directly from the various experts themselves, so I began to read their books. I also, viewed hours of online symposiums, tapings of large medical conferences, interviews, lectures, and talks. I read studies, articles, and research papers. I took notebooks full of notes. The more I learned, the more ferocious my appetite for more knowledge and information grew. I had no idea at the time that I would be writing a book.

This book came into being almost by happenstance. My brother was pressing me for a weight loss plan. At the time, I had no formal written plan because I had thrown it out. You see it was and still is, against my principles to use the methods I had originally been trained in, since I no longer had any faith in them. I was still in the middle of doing my research, and had postponed taking on any clients because I wanted to have my facts straight before I tried to help anyone. I told my brother that I wasn't done with my research, but he knew that I myself, had already begun to follow some of the principles which you will find later on in this book, and he asked me again for help. I agreed, but explained that some of the information might change as I continued to learn more. He was happy with the arrangement, so I began typing up some food lists and guidelines based on everything that I had already learned. I spent the whole afternoon typing. I was amazed by just how much information there was to convey. I couldn't help but think, my god it's like writing a book!

Shazam! The lightning struck. I could write a book!

I have always wanted to make a positive contribution to the world, to do something meaningful that would help others. In the past, I'd often wondered how I could accomplish this. Now, I had finally found a way. I could take all of my hours of reading, and research, and all of the information that I had gathered and sifted through, and share my conclusions with you. I could save you, and many others, the time and expense, and share with you the answers. I could help so many people. Right then and there, I decided to write this book!

I believe that everyone deserves a chance to live a life free from the burdens and suffering that come with chronic illness. In these pages, I will share with you, how to improve your overall health, reduce your risks for chronic disease, and how to lose weight and/or maintain a healthy body weight. When you have reached the end of this book, you will know exactly what to do, what to eat, and what not to eat. You'll understand how to become the healthiest, best version of yourself and you'll have the knowledge to help you enjoy this kind of wellbeing for the rest of your life.

CHAPTER 1

THE PROBLEM

A s I STATED EARLIER, there has recently been an abundance of emerging information from the scientific and medical communities, which points to a direct connection between what we eat, what we do, and how we feel. Nutrition and lifestyle have been found to be major players in a long list of illnesses, diseases, and disorders. These include, but are not limited to: alopecia, Alzheimer's, arteriosclerosis, autism spectrum disorder, cancer, chronic fatigue syndrome, cirrhosis of the liver, diabetes mellitus type 2, depression, food sensitivities, gastroesophageal reflux disease, gout, heart disease, hypertension, inflammatory bowel disease, obesity, and arthritis.

In 2014, the Journal of the American Medical Association reported that 34.5% of adults and 17% of youths in America were obese. Obesity is directly related to an increased risk for diabetes mellitus type 2, heart disease, cancer, high blood pressure, and sleep apnea. According to the CDC, heart disease is the leading cause of death in America. Each year approx. 610,000 people die from cardiovascular disease in the U.S.A.

Over 29 million Americans have diabetes. Per the American Diabetes Association, diabetes was the seventh leading cause of death in the United States in 2010, and diabetes was mentioned as a cause of death in a total of 234,051 death certificates. While these numbers alone should be enough to underline the serious nature of this disease, a newer 2017 study, published in the journal PLoS ONE, found that diabetes was actually the third leading cause of death in America, and not the seventh as had been previously believed.

These facts don't even take into account the rest of the world, but metabolic syndrome is quickly becoming a worldwide health epidemic. Metabolic syndrome is a combination of factors that increase a person's risk for heart disease, diabetes, and stroke. Such factors include high triglyceride levels, low HDL levels, high blood pressure, high blood sugar levels, insulin resistance, and obesity.

As reported by the World Health Organization, in 2014, more than 1.9 billion adults 18 years and older were overweight. Of these, over 600 million were obese. This equates to 39% of the world's adults being overweight, and 13% being obese. So in 2014, an astonishing 52% of the world's population were overweight or obese. Since 1980 worldwide obesity has more than doubled!

The worst news is that this rising obesity rate is no longer only an adult problem. In 2013, 42 million children under the age of 5 were overweight or obese, and per the CDC, childhood obesity in America has more than doubled in children, and quadrupled in adolescents, over the past 30 years. This means the health and wellbeing of our children is also in jeopardy.

WHAT'S IT TO ME?

My maternal grandparents were two of the most wonderful people you could ever come across. Wherever they went in the world, they made lifelong friends. It seemed like anyone who met them couldn't help but fall in love with them both. They used to get letters, postcards, and even occasionally gifts from people they'd met, who lived all over the world. They were kind, and warm hearted.

My childhood memories are full of my Nanny and the wonderful stories that she would make up to tell me. She would knit and crochet hats, vests, and sweaters for me and my siblings. She was a wonderful cook, and her home always smelled like good things cooking. She was a worry wart who didn't let me stand too close to the curb, or stand in more than half an inch of water at the beach! I adored her. I often joke that I inherited the "worry gene" from her.

My memories of her also include the special diet, which she would occasionally cheat on, for her type 2 diabetes, and that she had to take nitroglycerin for her angina. She was always a little overweight, and her arms were usually cool on my face, when I pressed my cheek to her on a hot summer day. I don't know every medical condition that she had, but I do remember that at one point she was taking so many different medications that she could barely walk in a straight line, even with assistance.

My grandfather, who we lovingly called Poppy, was the patriarch. He took so much pride in the generations that he and my grandmother started together. He was a hard worker and a family man. He was extremely intelligent, with a devilishly good sense of humor. He didn't own a car, and he used to walk everywhere. He used to take me on long walks with him to the park, the movies, and to the grocery stores and shops in his neighborhood. He ate yogurt with his breakfast almost every day. He loved fresh fruit, and salads with mayonnaise for salad dressing. He used to always tell me, "everything in moderation." He was relatively healthy for most of his long life. He did develop prostate cancer late in life, and very late in life he was diagnosed with type 2 diabetes and a slow growing form of bone cancer. He died at 93 from pneumonia.

I never knew my paternal grandparents. They died before I was born. My grandmother Anna died of cancer at age 58. My grandfather Robert died at 47 from sudden cardiac arrest.

My father. My childhood hero and protector. As a little girl, I remember that my dad seemed like a mountain to me, at six feet tall. Due to my fear of the dentist, my dad was the only one I would allow to take me to appointments. Upon arrival, I would immediately announce a need to use the restroom. My poor dad would routinely and patiently be forced to enter the girl's bathroom to retrieve me. If he did not, I would never have come out on my own. As a child, my dad taught me to swim and how to ride horses. He bought me my very first set of oil paints. Growing up, I spent many hours with him working on various projects, like cutting up the branches from a fallen tree, painting the inside walls of our home, and partnering on catering jobs together. He taught me that I could do anything that I put my mind to.

I almost lost the chance to share any of this with him, though. When my sister and I were just toddlers, a life-threatening form of cancer was discovered in his neck. Thanks to the work of a brilliant doctor, and a complex surgery, he made a full recovery. When I was a young teen, my dad was put on a salt-restricted diet, and began taking medication for high blood pressure. At one point, his pressure was so out of control; he was hospitalized. As the years went on, he had to overcome prostate cancer and, more recently, a thyroid removal surgery. To replace the hormones his body can no longer make for itself, he will be on hormone replacement therapy for the rest of his life.

My mom. Oh, the complicated relationship between a mother and a daughter. There is such a deep bond, and yet also the unique ability to drive each other completely mad. Of course, I have many lovely childhood memories of time spent with my mom, too. She always smelled like perfume, and I always thought she was beautiful beyond compare. We spent rainy afternoons together, playing board games or cards. She taught me to cook, bake, and garden; and she patiently tolerated the ensuing mess that came with all my creativity. For as long as I can remember, she has always been on one diet or another. She yo-yo dieted for most of my life. Big or small, I always thought she was more beautiful than any movie star. I remember how vibrant and active she used to be. She had a flourishing social life. She'd run around town with her girlfriends, going shopping, to the salon, and to luncheons. She was a great bowler, who played in a league, and she was very active in charity work.

She was diagnosed with type 2 diabetes in her early forties. At 75, she now suffers with the multitude of complications that inevitably come as your body is broken down by this disease. Like her mother before her, she is on a host of medications. Her poor health has left her housebound and she is rarely able to attend social events or family functions.

I also grew up with the sweet, happy, and sometimes mischievous girl that was my sister Robin. Robin was always a part of my life, as she was my senior by three years. At three years, old Robin was diagnosed with having an emotional disability. It was over fifty years ago, and not very much was known about autism spectrum disorder back then. Sometimes, pervasive thinking, false beliefs, or lack of knowledge can lead even well-meaning physicians to give out bad advice. The doctors at that time told my parents that Robin was deaf, couldn't see very well, would never speak or feed herself, and would require more care than my parents could possibly give to her. They advised my parents to place her into a home, for the good of all involved. You see, back then it was also considered a shameful secret to have a disabled child. My family was almost torn apart as other family members chimed in, agreeing with the doctor's advice. Despite everything, my parents loved their baby too much to give her up. Not knowing, at the time, how wrong the doctor's proclamations would be, they kept her anyway. She learned to speak, to feed herself, to walk, to climb, and to run. She had unimaginable energy, and she was at times way more than a handful, for sure. She had laser sharp vision, and not only could she hear, she had an uncanny ear for music. It wasn't long after her initial diagnosis that my parents found her humming along to music by Beethoven, which was playing on the radio!

As she grew up, she gave incredible joy to our family. She was always singing and laughing. Her happy spirit was contagious. It was impossible to be in a bad mood when she was happy. She had boundless love to give to her family, and to anyone else she came to know. She held no prejudices, she had no malice for anyone, and she had my grandfather's wickedly sharp sense of humor. She did have her limitations, and problems. Sometimes she could get very frustrated. She would repeat things over and over again. Sometimes it just seemed like an attempt to make conversation, but at other times, it seemed like she just couldn't get out what she really was trying to say. She would pull on her own hair, and cry with frustration. She was never able to have what most would call a normal life. She never left home, went to college, got a job, or found her soul mate. She suffered from skin rashes, food sensitivities, and alopecia, but overall Robin lived a happy existence. She was safe and secure; loved and accepted.

Robin passed away suddenly, in 2015. It was on July 4th, and for me, the fireworks that night were in tribute to her. It was just a short time before her 54th birthday, which would have been in August. She had barely shown signs of having anything more serious than a bad flu in the weeks before she went to the hospital. Once she was hospitalized, we were told by the doctors that she had pervasive amounts of cancer in her abdomen. The cancer had caused so many complications that treatment was not possible. She died in the hospital within 3 days.

Robin taught me the meaning of love. She taught me to have compassion, empathy, and patience for the differences in others. She lived her life with exuberance, every day. She loved people for their merit, and didn't concern herself with color, creed, or sexual orientation. Her sudden death made me realize that tomorrow could be a day too late, and that I needed to stop procrastinating, and go after my dreams today. My sister inspired me in life, and in death. The unique things that I learned from Robin will stay with me for the rest of my life.

My father-in-law, Ike, died of colon cancer at the age of 61. He was a good man. Not unlike my father and my grandfather, he, too, was a hard worker who loved his family, doted on his grandchildren, and was loyal to his friends. He was funny, kind, and generous.

My brother-in-law Barry had heart disease. He passed away two years ago, due to complications from cancer. He was only 62 years old. Barry was a devoted family man. He left behind three children, a grandson, and his wife of over 40 years. His family feels his loss daily.

My amazing mother-in-law, Selma, has been my best friend and confidant for more than 29 years. Selma is fighting a battle with cirrhosis of the liver. Oddly, she has never really been much of a drinker. She's a beautiful person who has always maintained a positive outlook on life. Over the years, she has repeatedly been there for us. She's been my cheerleader, my co-conspirator, and the voice of reason whenever I needed one. I love her very much. I admire her greatly for her grace, strength, and spirit.

There are several others, people who I count among my friends and family, who also suffer from chronic illness and disease.

I have been fortunate in that, somehow, I have thus far evaded any serious illness. I've spent much of my life battling with my own body weight. I was dieting by the time I was 14 or 15 years old. I have been rail thin, and I have been very overweight. My relationship with the scale, and with food, has been an unhealthy one. My turning point came about 4 years ago.

My husband, myself, and my daughter were living a distance away from family at the time. It was a good five-hour drive to see any of them. Back then, I was employed as a manager for a large wholesale and distribution chain. I was working 6 or 7 days a week, for 12 to 14 hours a day. My position in the company had no growth potential. I felt underappreciated, uninspired, and stressed out. I was about 30 pounds overweight. Being only five feet tall, thirty pounds is a lot of extra weight to carry. I was tired all the time, and I was miserable.

In the meanwhile, every time I spoke with my mom, dad, or brother on the phone, I was reminded of how poor my mother's health was. Over time, she consistently began to have new symptoms; her health issues seemed to become more and more complicated. Those phone conversations were my wake-up calls. Even back then, I understood that a person's weight and lifestyle could have a serious impact on their current and future health. I realized that I would have to make some big, permanent changes in my life if I wanted to avoid all the health issues that plagued my mother, and her mother before her.

My life, and the lives of so many others, have been touched by the diseases that afflict today's humanity. I believe we are facing the beginning of a worldwide health crisis.

My interest in this topic was initially sparked by my desire to avoid developing chronic illness, and to achieve optimal health for both myself, and my family. Realizing, now, that this situation is so much bigger than my own family, I would also like to do the same for you, and your family.

THE FACTS

Since the 1980's, obesity worldwide has more than doubled. Most of the world's population lives in countries where being overweight or obese kills more people than being underweight.

Some common health problems associated with adiposity (being overweight or obese) are cardiovascular diseases, diabetes, musculoskeletal disorders, and cancers like endometrial, breast, and colon. Cardiovascular diseases, chronic kidney disease, and diabetes are among leading global and regional causes of death. Between 1990 and 2010, the total number of deaths caused by cardiovascular diseases increased by more than 25%, and those of chronic kidney disease and diabetes nearly doubled. The number of people with diabetes has risen from 108 million, in 1980, to 422 million in 2014. Diabetes is a major cause of blindness, kidney failure, heart attacks, stroke, and lower limb amputation. Alzheimer's disease and cancers, such as liver cancer and pancreatic cancer, have also been linked to insulin resistance or diabetes. Almost half of all deaths attributable to high blood glucose occur before the age of 70 years. The

World Health Organization projects that diabetes will be the 7th leading cause of death, worldwide, in 2030.

Here are some interesting facts, put out by the National Health Council in 2014.

» Chronic diseases affect approximately 133 million Americans. By 2020, that number is expected to grow to an estimated 157 million, with 81 million having multiple conditions.

» Approximately one in two adults has a chronic condition.

» Approximately 8% of children, ages 5 to 17, were reported, by their parents, to have at least one chronic disease or disability.

» Many people suffer from more than one chronic illness.

» Almost a third of the population is now living with multiple chronic conditions.

» In 2009, seven in ten deaths in the U.S. were due to chronic diseases.

Clearly there is a common thread here. With the climbing obesity rate over the last 30 or so years, we are also experiencing an overwhelming surge in chronic illnesses. It's also important to note that chronic disease is not limited solely to those who are overweight. There are plenty of slim, seemingly healthy people, walking around with chronic illnesses. These illnesses run the gamut, and include everything from acid reflux disease to diabetes and cirrhosis of the liver. The reality is there are many people walking around today, undiagnosed, who don't even realize that they're sick.

CHAPTER 2

EPIC TALE OR EPIC FAIL?

So, WHAT'S GOING ON? Why are so many people overweight? Why are so many people sick?

Let me start by saying, that although the answers are definitely - diet and life style related, we are not overweight or sick because we somehow failed as individuals. The problem has nothing to do with self-indulgence, willpower, or laziness. Nobody I know wants to be overweight or sick. No parent would choose that for their kids either. The real answers are complicated. I will try to break them down for you as best as I can.

THE FIRST LAW, THE FIRST PROBLEM

The first problem is one we have had for a long time. It's in how we've come to view weight gain, and weight loss in the first place.

When I studied for my certifications to become a Personal Trainer, Weight Management Specialist, and Physique and Figure Training Specialist, I was taught that we gain weight because we eat too much and move to little. The course work illustrated among other things, that because of our busy lifestyles, people today often had no time to cook at home. This in turn, caused people to eat too much junk food and fast food. It also described how our technology filled lives, had left us sedentary. I was taught, that to help people lose weight and be healthier, I would have to educate them on how to eat less, make better food choices, and exercise more. Basically, it was up to me as a trainer and coach to set them straight. I must admit for a while I bought the whole argument. It supported everything I'd learned over the years. This was an accredited school with a great reputation, they must know what they were talking about, right?

Robert H. Lustig, M.D. is a Neuroendocrinologist. He also serves as Professor of Pediatrics in the Division of Endocrinology at University of California, San Francisco, and the Director of the Weight Assessment for Teen and Child Health (WATCH) Program at UCSF. In his 2013 book, Fat Chance, he wrote, "*To blame obesity on the obese is the easy answer, but it is the **wrong** answer. The current formulation of gluttony and sloth, diet and exercise, while accepted by virtually everyone, is based on faulty premises and myths that have taken hold in the world's consciousness.*"

My educators had based their literature and teachings, on this same formulation of gluttony and sloth, diet, and exercise. These concepts are so generally accepted; doctors and health organizations alike have been basing their recommendations on them for years. For example, the American cancer society has a chart on their web page which is titled, Make Exercise Work for You, which illustrates you how much exercise you'd have to do to work off a large order of fries, (see figure 1),

TO BURN OFF A LARGE ORDER OF FRIES (400 CALORIES)

A 160-pound person could burn off 400 calories in the time and activities shown below:

Activity	Minutes
Moderate walking	95
Scrubbing Floors	89
Dancing	70
Bicycling	39
Running	28

(Figure 1)

And according to a January 2016, on line article by The American Heart Association, you should follow the following advice,

» *"If you are trying not to gain weight, don't eat more calories than you know you can burn up every day."*

» *"Increase the amount and intensity of your physical activity to match the number of calories you take in."*

» *"Aim for at least 150 minutes of moderate physical activity or 75 minutes of vigorous physical activity – or an equal combination of both – each week."*

These pervasive, yet incorrect, concepts all hinge on something in physics called the first law of thermodynamics.

The first law of thermodynamics states, that the total energy of an isolated system is constant; energy can be transformed from one form to another, but cannot be created or destroyed. In other words, the body can neither, create nor destroy energy. It can only transfer energy from one state to another. So, when you take in energy in the form of food, it must be transferred to the muscles, organs, and tissues, where it will be used as energy. Excess energy will be stored as fat.

Based on this interpretation, if you expend more energy than you take in you will lose weight. No matter what you eat, if you consume less calories than you expend, you will burn fat and lose weight. While this all sounds very reasonable, it's an over simplification of the process.

FOOD IS MORE THAN SUSTENANCE

Let's begin our discussion by dispelling the notion that all calories are created equal. Everything we eat is processed by our bodies, but not everything we eat is processed in the same way.

Dr. Mark Hyman serves as chairman of the board for the Institute for Functional Medicine. He founded both The UltraWellness Center (located in Lenox, MA) and The Cleveland Clinic Center for Functional Medicine, which is located in Cleveland, OH.

In his book "Eat Fat, Get Thin", Dr. Hyman explains how our weight is affected by the types of foods we eat, and the biological responses those foods trigger. He wrote, *"This hormonal or metabolic hypothesis of weight gain supports the idea that it is the composition and quality of the foods you eat (and the hormones and biochemistry they subsequently trigger) that determine whether you lose or gain weight. In other words, **it is not how much you eat but what you eat** that controls the metabolic switches. Foods inherent information-the messages and instructions it contains is what drives your metabolism"*

What does that mean? It means that different foods interact with our systems in distinct ways. Food is more than sustenance. The quality of the foods we eat have a huge impact on our bodies and our health!

Foods are categorized into the following three macronutrients: carbohydrates, fats, and protein. These are then broken down even further within their categories, for example: carbohydrates can be starches, sugars, or fiber. Fats can be saturated, unsaturated, and mono-unsaturated. Proteins are either complete (containing all 22 amino acids), or incomplete. Essential (can't be synthesized by the body), non-essential, or conditional (needed in times of illness and stress).

Any food that is not a fat or a protein is a carbohydrate. Carbohydrates are not essential nutrients. There is no daily required amount of carbs. Refined carbohydrates tend to go through the digestion process very quickly, spiking our blood sugar levels and causing our bodies to respond by releasing insulin into the blood. Too much insulin in our blood can cause a number of difficulties for us.

Without insulin, there is no fat storage. Normally when we eat, some insulin is secreted by the pancreas into the blood. As we digest, some of the energy from our food is used by the body, and some of it is stored as fat. When things are functioning correctly, the food energy that is stored as fat is only stored temporarily. Once the meal has been completely digested and there is no more glucose in the blood, the energy which was temporarily stored as fat, is released from the fat cells back into the blood stream for use.

Problems can occur when we eat too many carbohydrates, especially refined carbs, and sugars which cause large sugar and insulin spikes in our blood. When there is too much insulin in our blood almost all the energy from the food gets pushed into our fat cells for storage, and is locked there. Very little energy is made available to the body for usage. When the food is completely digested, none of the energy which was stored as fat is released back into the blood for use, causing a sugar crash. This lack of available energy in the blood, tells our brain that we are starving. The body responds to this starvation emergency in two ways, by slowing down our energy expenditure, and by producing hormones which signal hunger. This hunger drives our cravings for the quickest form of available energy, which is carbohydrates. This becomes a vicious cycle. The more carbs we eat, the hungrier we become. The hungrier we become, the more carbs we eat. Meanwhile insulin continues to push all the energy from our food into our fat cells making us fatter and fatter. This eventually puts our overly full fat cells into distress and they become inflamed. When our fat cells become inflamed they release proteins called cytokines into the blood. The presence of cytokines in the blood causes systemic low grade inflammation. Chronic inflammation of this nature has been associated with Alzheimer's, hypertension, heart disease, insulin resistance, diabetes, and other chronic illnesses. Too many insulin spikes over time can also lead to insulin resistance. Insulin resistance is a state in which the body becomes insensitive to, or unresponsive to insulin. In a state of insulin resistance, more and more insulin is needed to handle the sugar in our blood. When the pancreas can no longer produce enough insulin to handle the sugar in our blood, it is called diabetes. Developing Type 2 diabetes is akin to developing an intolerance to carbohydrates.

Diabetes is somewhat of a doorway disease because having diabetes opens the door to increased risk of heart disease, vascular disease, kidney disease, vision loss and amputations. Recently a study on diabetes was published in The Lancet. The study evaluated the impact of diabetes on a global scale. Researchers examined data collected from 200 countries, over the last 35 years. They found that diabetes and its complications account for more than 2 million deaths every year, and are the seventh leading causes of disability worldwide. Additionally, the Global cost of diabetes is now 825 billion dollars per year!

Diabetes has been prevalent in my family, particularly on my mother's side for generations, leading as far back as my great grandparents, and possibly further. I equate this to culture, genetics, and hardship. When I was a kid, my grandmother was famous for her red rice with peas, her fideos (a pasta dish), and her pot roast with potatoes. I remember my dad used to tease her about being the only person he knew who would serve rice, potatoes, pasta, and bread all in the same meal. Nanny would laugh and say it was the only way to stretch the meal, especially, back when my dad was dating my mother, because he could eat so much, and she and Poppy, could only afford to buy a little meat. I remember many weekends when she brought rice and potatoes to our house to share at family dinners. I'm certain that rice, potatoes, and bread, which have always been a lot cheaper than meat, were staples at my grandmother's table. My grandparents lived during tough economic times. My grandfather worked for a factory unloading trucks for a living. They raised three children, and helped care for extended family on my grandfather's modest salary. I believe they ate the way they did out of necessity, and because eating habits are learned from your family. Recipes and traditions are passed down through the generations.

Insulin resistance which leads to diabetes, can also cause other problems. When we need energy, a hormone called ghrelin is secreted. Ghrelin is the hunger hormone. It signals us to eat. When we've eaten enough, a hormone called leptin is secreted. Leptin is the satiety hormone. It signals us to stop eating. When the cycle is complete, we literally have energy to burn. However, when there is too much insulin in the blood, the insulin can block the leptin signal from getting to the brain. When this happens the person, who is insulin resistant, is now also leptin resistant. Even when the stomach is full the brain never gets the message to stop eating. A person who is leptin resistant can feel hungry all the time. The only effective way to reduce leptin resistance is by lowering the amount of insulin in the blood. To reduce the amount of insulin in the blood, you must avoid carbohydrates. Especially refined carbohydrates and sugar.

Sugar is a source of dangerous inflammation which has been linked to many chronic diseases like Alzheimer's, diabetes, hypertension, and cancer. Numerous studies have sited a correlation between Alzheimer's disease and diabetes.

In a 2016 article, published in the Journal of Alzheimer's Disease, New York University professor Melissa A. Schilling wrote, regarding her own investigations, "*The results suggest that avoiding excess insulin, and supporting robust IDE levels, could be important ways of preventing and lessening the impact of AD.*" (IDE refers to insulin-degrading enzyme, an enzyme which is secreted by cells to mitigate insulin in the blood)

In a study, which was published in 2002 in the Journal of the National Cancer Institute, researchers sought to investigate the relationship between high glycemic diets, post meal blood sugar spikes, and pancreatic cancer. It was a continuation of the famous 1976 Nurses' Health Study, a study which originally followed 121,700 nurses to research the potential long-term consequences of oral contraceptives. The new research studied 88,802 of the original participants from 1980-1984. Researchers expressed that insulin and insulin resistance may play a role in promoting pancreatic cancer. They concluded that although statistics did not support an overall association between dietary glycemic load and pancreatic cancer, there was a statistically significant influence of glycemic load on pancreatic cancer risk among overweight and sedentary individuals, and that this data supported the hypothesis that, "abnormal glucose metabolism and states of relative hyperinsulinemia enhance pancreatic carcinogenesis." In other words, being diabetic and having too much insulin in the blood increases the risks for pancreatic cancer.

In 2006, another large study was done and published, in the American Journal of Nutrition. This study examined the association of added sugar and of high-sugar foods with the risk of pancreatic cancer. The study followed 77,797 men and women for eight years. Data collected during this study supported researcher's hypothesis that a high consumption of sugar and sweetened foods may be associated with the risk of pancreatic cancer.

In July of 2009, Dr. Robert Lustig, in conjunction with the University of California presented, Sugar the Bitter Truth. It was a video presentation filmed as part of a series called, Mini Medical School for the Public. In his presentation, Dr. Lustig demonstrated how sugar, especially fructose (the kind of sugar found in high fructose corn syrup), is processed through our livers in exactly the same manner as alcohol. This is significant because it means that eating too much sugar can cause as much damage to your liver, as drinking too much alcohol.

Let me explain how it happens. Sugar is composed of glucose and fructose. Fructose and alcohol are both processed by the liver. If you think about it, alcohol is just sugar that's been fermented. The liver uses fructose to create fat. Given enough fructose, fat begins to accumulate in the liver. A buildup of fat in the liver causes a condition known as called Non-alcoholic fatty liver disease (NAFLD). 1 in 3 adults, and 1 in 10 children in America have NAFLD. Non-alcoholic fatty liver disease can become Non-alcoholic steatohepatitis (NASH).

NASH, is a very similar condition to alcoholic liver disease. In NASH, there is an accumulation of excess fat, inflammation, damage, and scarring, in the liver of people who drink little or no alcohol. NASH is often called silent liver disease, because it has almost no symptoms. The people who are affected by it often feel well, and are unaware that there's even a problem. NASH is very serious and can lead to cirrhosis of the liver. Astonishingly, you don't have to be a drinker to develop cirrhosis of the liver.

As reported by an article in the August 25, 2016 issue of the New England Journal of Medicine, cirrhosis is the 8th leading cause of death in the USA and the 13th leading cause of death globally, representing a 45.6% increase worldwide since 1990.

Due to the increasing prevalence of NAFLD, cirrhosis related to NASH is predicted to become the most common reason for orthotopic liver transplantation in the USA. Diagnosis often occurs after a liver enzyme test comes back a little elevated, but NAFLD can be present even with a normal liver blood test result. The best way to screen for NAFLD is with an ultrasound of the liver.

Think back to my mother-in-law Selma. She has Cirrhosis of the liver, yet she has never been much of a drinker. She has however, always loved her sweets. Jelly doughnuts and gooey ice cream sundaes with caramel sauce, have always been her favorites.

But even with her sweet tooth, Selma's daily dietary habits have pretty much been the same as the typical American diet. For breakfast, most days she'd have orange juice, coffee with sugar, white toast, and her favorite hot cereal (a package of instant maple & brown sugar oatmeal). On days when she was running late to work, she'd sometimes grab a breakfast sandwich at Mc Donald's. Lunches needed to be portable for work and often consisted of a juice box, a sandwich on white bread, a couple of low fat cookies, and a piece of fruit. A low-fat cereal bar, or a piece of white bread with a tiny smear of butter, would tide her over until dinner. Sweetened ice tea or soda were routinely served with dinner. Most nights there would be a few low-fat cookies, a thin slice of packaged cake, or a small piece of pie for dessert. As many of us do, she sometimes indulged in her favorite treats on the weekends, and she enjoyed some extra goodies around the holidays, and on birthdays.

Selma has been very careful over the years to maintain a healthy weight, and has always remained slim. In truth, she takes pride in having healthy habits. She has always been great about going for regular checkups, and health screenings, and she has diligently followed all the low fat and low cholesterol dietary recommendations made to her by both the USDA, and her personal physician. Could Selma's non-alcoholic cirrhosis be related to years of sugar consumption, refined carbohydrates, and processed foods which are notoriously loaded with high fructose corn syrup? There is strong scientific evidence which leads me to say yes.

While there is no daily requirement for carbohydrates, your body does require the nutrients found in fresh fruits, vegetables, and dark leafy greens. These unrefined types of carbohydrate foods contain phytonutrients, fiber, vitamins, and minerals which are needed by our bodies for function and health. We want to have an abundance of these incorporated into our daily dietary plan.

Phytonutrients and antioxidants, help prevent cancer by protecting our cells from the damaging effects of free radicals and oxidation. They can be found in colorful fruits and vegetables like: beets, dark leafy greens, blue berries, carrots, cherries, and tomatoes. Coffee, tea, red wine, and dark chocolate, also contain powerful antioxidants.

Foods like: apples, raspberries, asparagus, broccoli, and beans, are all high in fiber, which is an important dietary component. Fiber helps us to feel full, stay regular, and promotes good colon health. Fiber is also a favorite food of the beneficial bacteria which live in our intestines and help regulate our bodies. Fresh fruits and vegetables are also filled with essential vitamins and minerals needed for all sorts of biological processes like, cell growth, blood clotting, and energy.

Essential fatty acids (EFAs) are needed for optimal health but they can't be synthesized by the body, so they must be obtained through diet. Healthy fats like omega 3's and omega 9's are found in nuts, fatty fish, avocados, and olive oil. These fats promote healthy skin, hair, and nails. Additionally, they are anti-inflammatory, and help support vascular, heart, and brain health.

It's important to note, that nearly 60% of your brain is made up of fat. Fatty acids are critical to the brains function and integrity. In fact, studies have shown that eating a diet which is higher in fat can dramatically reduce the risks for dementia and Alzheimer's disease, while an imbalance in the dietary intake of fatty acids has been associated with impaired brain performance and disease.

Interestingly, while high sugar consumption has been associated with lower testosterone levels in men, eating a diet that is high in healthy fats, has been found to increase testosterone levels.

Fats help us feel full sooner than other foods, and they speed up our metabolism. Fats are more readily used for energy, and are less likely to be stored as fat in the body because, dietary fats have little to no effect on insulin secretion. Remember, without Insulin there is no fat storage.

As with carbohydrates, not all fats are created equally. While omega 3 and omega 9 fats are healthy and anti-inflammatory, eating certain refined oils and too many omega 6 fats, can cause unhealthy, dangerous inflammation. Certain oils should be avoided altogether these include: trans fats, hydrogenated oils, and refined oils. Vegetable oils like: soy, corn, canola, cotton seed, sunflower and safflower, are all refined oils. Refined oils have been treated with high temperatures, and caustic chemicals which make them an unhealthy option. Additionally, the over use of these inexpensive, refined oils by the food industry, has injected our diets with too many omega 6 fats.

Most omega 6 fats cause inflammation. Even so, a certain amount of omega 6's are needed for good health, and not all omega 6 fats are harmful.

The ideal ratio is 1-1. In the common western diet however, the ratio is closer to 16 to 1, with the amount of Omega 3's being severely deficient. This imbalance promotes the pathogenesis of many diseases including: cardiovascular disease, cancer, inflammatory disease, and autoimmune diseases. Increased amounts of omega 3's with decreased amounts omega 6's (lower omega 6/ omega 3 ratios) have been proven to suppress these kinds of illnesses. As stated in a 2008 article, by Artemis Simopoulos, the founder and president of the Center for Genetics, Nutrition, and Health, "*In the secondary prevention of cardiovascular disease, a ratio of 4/1 was associated with a 70% decrease in total mortality. A ratio of 2.5/1 reduced rectal cell proliferation in patients with colorectal cancer, whereas a ratio of 4/1 with the same amount of omega-3 PUFA had no effect. The lower omega-6/omega-3 ratio in women with breast cancer was associated with decreased risk. A ratio of 2-3/1 suppressed inflammation in patients with rheumatoid arthritis, and a ratio of 5/1 had a beneficial effect on patients with asthma, whereas a ratio of 10/1 had adverse consequences. These studies indicate that the optimal ratio may vary with the disease under consideration. This is consistent with the fact that chronic diseases are multigenic and multifactorial.*"

The bottom line is, a lower ratio of omega 6/omega 3 fatty acids reduces the risk for many of the chronic diseases which are prevalent today.

Proteins are found in every cell of the body. They're required for structure, function, and the regulation of tissues and organs. The body uses protein to make enzymes, hormones, and other body chemicals. Protein is an important building block of bones, muscles, cartilage, skin, and blood. The body does not store protein, and therefore has no reservoir to draw on when it needs a new supply. Therefore, having the right amount of quality proteins in your diet is so important. Depending on age and activity level, 10-35% of a person's diet should consist of protein.

High protein diets, where protein makes up more than 35% of the dietary intake, have been associated with: nausea, diarrhea, and hyperinsulinemia, a condition in which there are excess levels of insulin circulating in the blood relative to the level of glucose. Hyperinsulinemia is one of the symptoms of pre-diabetes which leads to insulin resistance. There are also concerns that, eating too much protein may cause a buildup of urea nitrogen in the blood exceeding the livers ability to process it. Evidence also suggests a relationship between high-protein intake, prostate cancer, and renal cell cancer.

A diet which is high in refined carbohydrates, refined oils, sugar, and red meat is an inflammatory diet, which can lead to chronic inflammation in the body. Dietary items such as garlic, dark leafy greens, olive oil, and turmeric are all anti-inflammatory foods, which reduce inflammation. (See figure 2 for a more comprehensive list.) Chronic Inflammation is not only associated with chronic diseases; it has also been linked to certain cancers.

Inflammatory foods	Anti-inflammatory foods
Trans fats	Berries
White Bread	Nuts & Seeds
White Rice	Whole Grains
French Fries and Fried Foods	Dark Leafy Greens
Soda	Mushrooms
Sugar and Corn syrup	Hot and Sweet Peppers
Omega 6 Fatty Acids	Omega 3 Fatty Acids
Mono sodium glutamate (MSG)	Tomatoes
Gluten	Beets
Dairy	Carrots, Parsnips & Turnips
Alcohol	Zucchini and Cucumbers
	Tart Cherries
	Black Pepper
	Ginger & Turmeric
	Garlic & Onions
	Cocoa & Dark Chocolate
	Basil, Rosemary, dill, Thyme & other Herbs
	Cruciferous Vegetables
	Avocado

(Figure 2)

I would like to tell you a little bit more about my father-in-law Ike. Sadly, he passed away over 25 years ago, at the young age of 61 from colon cancer. Ike was a wonderful man. He worked as a bell captain and concierge for a fine hotel in Manhattan. His job kept him busy, and could be very stressful at times. He was friendly, outgoing, and he loved to play golf with his friends on his days off. He was handsome, slim, and full of energy. He had a great sense of humor, and he was surprisingly generous. Ike would have given you the shirt from his back if he thought you were in need. His generosity was only surprising, if you knew that he had been born just a few short months before the beginning of the Great Depression, into a family where he was just one out of fourteen other children. Growing up he never had much, and probably had to share quite a bit. These were very hard times, and it's likely that Ike wasn't exposed to very many fresh fruits or vegetables as he grew up.

When he became a man his adult tastes, through no fault of his own, were limited by the scarcity he'd experienced in his childhood. He wasn't accustomed to foods that had many spices in them, and so he liked his food to remain fairly plain. He only ate a small variety of vegetables, which included: corn, peas & carrots, cucumber, canned green beans, and tomatoes. He never ate things like: Brussels sprouts, broccoli, cauliflower, garlic, eggplant, avocado, leafy greens, onions, or squash, and except for the occasional banana, he didn't eat much fruit either. Hamburgers with mashed potatoes and peas, a broiled steak with some french fries and a tossed salad, and meatball subs from the pizza place down the block were some of Ike's favorite meals. He would periodically eat some chicken, but not much fish. The lettuce in his salad was always iceberg. He ate white bread, and drank coffee, sweetened iced tea, and soda. He loved candy, pretzels, popcorn, and potato chips. His living room coffee table was always loaded up with a variety of these kinds of treats.

As a young man, Ike had become a smoker. Though he had tried many times, he was never able to quit. Every evening after dinner, he would retire to his favorite chair in the living room to unwind from the stresses of the day. He would relax with a cold beer, while he snacked in front of the television, and smoked his cigarettes.

Though he was very physically active, Ike didn't live a very healthy lifestyle. He was never given the tools to manage the stresses of daily life. He worked a difficult and often hectic job. As many people do, Ike tried to relieve his tension with junk food, a cold beer, and a pack of cigarettes. Additionally, Ike's regular diet was highly inflammatory, and almost devoid of any phytonutrients, or antioxidants. It was also, very low in fiber, high in sugar, and high in refined carbohydrates. His lifestyle and diet where important contributing factors in the disintegration of his health, and his early death.

The quality of the foods we eat, have an undeniable impact on our health, our weight, and on our mortality. Foods trigger hormonal and biological responses. Foods can cause, or mitigate inflammation. The foods we eat can boost our health or steal it away from us.

Dr. David Ludwig is a highly-regarded endocrinologist, researcher, and professor at Harvard Medical School. He is also the director of the New Balance Foundation Obesity Prevention Center at Boston Children's Hospital. He has spent years researching how food affects hormones, body weight and well-being.

In his 2016 book, Always Hungry, Dr. Ludwig wrote, "*After every meal, hormones, chemical reactions, and even the activity of genes throughout the body change in radically different ways, all according to what we eat. These biological effects of food, quite apart from calorie content, could make all the difference between feeling persistently hungry or satisfied, between having low or robust energy, between weight gain or loss, and between a lifetime of chronic disease or one of good health.*" To sum it up, a calorie is not, just a calorie.

CHAPTER 3

SCRATCH THAT, REVERSE IT!

Now that we've established that a calorie is not just a calorie, let's address this whole issue of gluttony and sloth. We've all had it drummed into us to eat less and move more. We've all been conditioned to believe that if we eat, we'd better burn off the calories or they'll be stored as fat. This whole concept is backwards, here's why:

When everything in the body is functioning normally, we eat to get the energy we need. We're active when we have the energy to burn. When we don't eat enough calories, we physically don't have the energy to expend. When this happens, the body reacts by dialing back our metabolism, leaving us feeling lethargic, and turning us into couch potatoes.

Our bodies are biological wonders, which are internally regulated. Each of us has an inherent bodyweight set point. Think of it as something like a thermostat that controls your weight. Your body always naturally works to return to that setting/weight.

Dr. Gerard E. Mullin, MD, is an associate professor in the department of medicine, and the director of Integrative Gastroenterology Nutrition Services at the Johns Hopkins Hospital. He is also a recipient of the Grace A. Goldsmith award for achievement in the field of nutrition.

In his recent book, *The Gut Balance Revolution*, he explains, "*Calories in/calories out doesn't work for the masses, because it can't work. It can't work, because simply reducing the amount of food you consume and spending more energy exercising doesn't necessarily influence your body weight set point."*

When we restrict our food intake and ignore hunger cues, continue to eat even though we feel full, or have lunch just because the clock on the wall says it's lunch time, we are interfering with that biological thermostat. It's for this reason that people who practice mindful eating (eating in accordance with their bodies natural hunger and satiety cues,) tend to maintain a more stable bodyweight and metabolism than those who do not.

Dieting is a sure-fire way to slow your metabolism, and yo-yo dieting could result in an even higher bodyweight set point. Due to biological mechanisms meant to defend against starvation, when you diet, your body will fight against your efforts to lose weight. To protect itself, the body will ramp up hunger signals and cravings, while conserving as much energy as possible. It will fiercely hang on to any calories taken in, making weight loss very difficult. This is known as the starvation response, and even if you succeed in losing weight, much of your weight loss efforts will be in vain. As soon as you stop dieting, your body will respond by attempting to return to the weight set point, and you will begin to gain back the weight.

It won't be your fault; it's biology working against you. You can't win this game, because nature has rigged it. One of the lasting effects of dieting is a slower metabolism. Your post-diet body will burn less daily calories now, than it did before. On top of everything else, your bodyweight set point could be raised by the yo-yo effects of dieting. When it's all over and done, you could easily end up weighing more than you did before you started!

In August of 2016, a study was published by the journal *Obesity*, which conclusively proved this very thing. The Biggest Loser is a television program, which first aired on NBC in 2004. On the show, contestants compete to lose weight by following a program of rigid calorie restriction, in combination with hours of extreme physical activity. In the study, researchers followed former contestants of the television program for a period of six years after they had left the show. The results were astounding! Newspapers, magazines, and television networks across the country reported on the study.

Researchers found that in the years following their last appearances on the show, most of the contestants had gained back significant amounts of the weight they had lost, and they had also experienced a colossal slowdown of their metabolisms.

It's not uncommon for a person's metabolic rate to be slower than usual directly after being on a calorie-restricted diet. The incredible part was that these people's metabolisms had never recovered! Over the years, their resting metabolic rates (RMRs) had gotten slower and slower. Per the study's authors, *"The Biggest Loser" participants with the greatest weight loss at the end of the competition also experienced the greatest slowing of RMR at that time. Similarly, those who were most successful at maintaining lost weight after 6 years also experienced greater ongoing metabolic slowing."*

Six years later, participants' average daily resting metabolic rates were 500 calories lower than expected for people of their age and body composition! The New York Times reported that season 8's winner Danny Cahill currently eats 800 calories a day less than a typical man of his size. If he eats anything more, it gets stored as fat.

The scientists involved in this study concluded, *"Therefore, long-term weight loss requires vigilant combat against persistent metabolic adaptation that acts to proportionally counter ongoing efforts to reduce body weight."*

To put it in a nut shell, these people ate a lot less, and moved a lot more. Their bodies were left so traumatized that six years later, they're still reacting. Over time, these people will be forced to eat fewer and fewer calories to avoid having them stored as fat.

Nature has rigged the game in an effort to protect the body from times of scarcity. The lasting effects of dieting are a slower metabolism, increased hunger, and a return to the original body weight set point, or a new higher one. So much for eat less and move more!

GLUTTONY AND SLOTH

Dr. Benjamin Caballero is a professor of international health and of pediatrics, and is the director of the Center for Human Nutrition at the Schools of Public Health and of Medicine, John Hopkins University. He is also a member of the Food and Nutrition Board of the Nutrition Institute of Medicine, National Academy of Sciences, and of the Nutrition and Metabolism Study Section, National Institutes of Health. He specializes in the areas of childhood nutrition, and obesity in minorities and developing country populations.

In 2005, he wrote an article in The New England Journal of Medicine. It was called "A Nutrition Paradox-Underweight and Obesity in Developing Countries." In it, he spoke of his experiences in a primary care clinic which was located in the slums of Sao Paulo, Brazil. *"The waiting room was full of mothers with thin, stunted young children, exhibiting the typical signs of chronic undernutrition. Their appearance, sadly would surprise few who visit poor urban areas in the developing world. What might come as a surprise is that many of the mothers holding those undernourished infants were themselves overweight."*

He attributed this surprising paradox to the poverty of the area. He believed that the least expensive foods were also the least nutritious. He surmised that the mothers were overweight, while the babies were underdeveloped and thin, due to the poor quality of their food. The babies were underweight, not because their mothers ate too much food or didn't feed them enough, but because children require much higher amounts of vitamins and nutrients than adults. Simply put, the children weren't getting enough nutrition from the food they ate-- nutrition which they needed to develop and thrive.

In this same article, Dr. Caballero also wrote about a phenomenon he called "fetal Origins of disease." *"The hypothesis of "fetal Origins of disease," which is supported by a number of observational epidemiologic studies, postulates that early (intrauterine or early postnatal) undernutrition causes an irreversible differentiation of metabolic systems, which may, in turn increase the risks of certain chronic diseases in adulthood. For example, a fetus of an undernourished mother will respond to a reduced energy supply by switching on genes that optimize energy conservation. This survival strategy causes a permanent differentiation of regulatory systems that result in an excess accumulation of energy (and consequently of body fat) when the adult is exposed to an unrestricted dietary energy supply. Because intrauterine growth retardation and low birth weight are common in developing countries, this mechanism may result in the establishment of a population in which many adults are particularly susceptible to becoming obese."*

So, in essence, these people were undernourished, and suffering from malnutrition which began intrauterine, or before they were even born. The very scarcity they were born into is the explanation for the obesity they suffered when they became adults. The mothers were overweight due to the low quality of the available foods, the starvation response, and intrauterine undernutrition.

In his article, Dr. Caballero clearly illustrated the influence that a diet lacking in nutrition can have on our weight, our health, our biological functions, and our genes. He shows us, through his experiences in Sao Paulo, that undernourished, starving people can still be overweight. Thus, dispelling the myth of gluttony and sloth.

HORMONES, LIFESTYLE, AND OTHER CONSIDERATIONS

We've already discussed some of the ways that insulin can affect our fat cells and our health. Other hormones, like estrogen, testosterone, and cortisol, can also play a role. Obesity and hormonal imbalances often go hand in hand.

ESTROGEN AND TESTOSTERONE

Too much or too little estrogen or testosterone can cause all kinds of physical and emotional discomforts. An excess of estrogen in men can lead to dropping testosterone levels, lowered sex drive, sexual dysfunction, and weight gain. In women, excess estrogen levels can cause weight gain, headaches, fatigue, mood swings, and abnormal menstrual cycles. Eating a nutrient dense diet, with plenty of healthy fats, can help restore hormonal balance.

STRESS AND CORTISOL

Cortisol is a hormone released into the bloodstream during times of stress. It's the hormone responsible for many of the physiological responses that take place in the body during times of imminent danger. The release of cortisol increases sugars in the bloodstream, and enhances the brain's use of glucose. It also curbs nonessential functions, helping us react quickly to survive during a fight-or-flight situation. Normally, this response is temporary, and quickly recedes after the danger has past. Living in states of constant stress can cause cortisol to remain in the bloodstream. Overexposure to cortisol, and other stress related hormones, causes the storage of belly fat, and puts us at increased risk for many serious concerns, such as depression, weight gain, sleep disorders, memory impairment, digestive issues, cancer, hypertension, type 2 diabetes, and stroke. If that wasn't bad enough, too much belly fat often equates to too much estrogen, since the fat cells in belly fat produce estrogen. Stress is an important component of the lifestyle and environmental factors that can impact our well-being, and must be managed. Another equally important component is sleep.

GETTING YOUR ZZZ'S

Getting a good night's sleep may be more meaningful than you realize. Studies have shown that even modest sleep disturbances impair our thinking and our motor skills. (Think about how this could affect someone operating heavy machinery or driving a car). Moderate sleep disturbances also increase the secretion of pro-inflammatory cytokines. If you recall, cytokines are proteins that cause the inflammation associated with heart disease, Alzheimer's, and diabetes. Chronic sleep restriction has been linked to insulin resistance, lower levels of leptin (the satiety hormone,) and higher levels of ghrelin (the hunger hormone.)

In a 2011 European study, healthy men were deprived of sleep for 24 hours. The sleep-deprived men reported experiencing magnified feelings of hunger. Additionally, when they were shown pictures of food, they had increased activity in a part of the brain that connects food with pleasure and reward. The tired men also tended to choose higher calorie foods over lower calorie foods when given a choice.

In a more recent, 2014 study, funded by the Mayo Clinic, researchers studied healthy people ages 18-40, and found that moderate sleep restriction causes endothelial dysfunction. The endothelium is a thin membrane that lines the inside of the heart and blood vessels. Endothelial cells release substances that control vascular relaxation and contraction. They also release enzymes that control blood clotting, blood flow, and immune function. Endothelial dysfunction can interfere with arteries' ability to dilate, and it can also cause atherosclerosis (a chronic disease characterized by the thickening and hardening of the arteries,) thereby significantly increasing the risk of heart attack and stroke. Endothelial dysfunction is usually caused by high blood pressure, diabetes, and smoking.

In the study, which was published in the Journal of the American Heart Association, researchers affirmed, "*We found that moderate sleep restriction during an 8-day period is associated with a significant impairment in flow-mediated vasodilatation. The magnitude of impairment seen in this study with sleep restriction is similar to that reported in people who smoke, or have diabetes, or who have coronary artery disease, and helps further our understanding of the cardiovascular risks association with sleep deprivation. The potential public health impact of this relationship may be enormous given the high prevalence of voluntary sleep restriction."*

In summary, moderate sleep restriction causes enhanced hunger, which can lead to weight gain. It also increases the risk for injury and chronic illnesses like diabetes, heart attack, stroke, and mortality. This means that getting enough sleep is a crucial element of good health.

THE BODY IN MOTION: USE IT OR LOSE IT

Being able to enjoy an evening stroll with your honey, or a bike ride in the park with your kids, is a precious gift. Unfortunately for some, having the strength to walk to the bathroom without assistance, or having the dignity of getting dressed on their own, would also be a gift.

Our bodies were made to be in motion. Have you ever heard of Newton's first law of motion? It states that an object at rest stays at rest and an object in motion stays in motion. This is true of the body as well. A prolonged lack of physical activity causes the heart and lungs to weaken, while the muscles begin to atrophy. I have witnessed in my own family, how a sedentary lifestyle can slowly dismantle a person's health. Even a healthy, young individual will lose muscle strength and physical capacity if they remain inactive for too long, but the risks go beyond that.

On April 4[th,] 2002, the World Health Organization issued a warning against the dangers of physical inactivity. They warned that approximately 2 million deaths per year are attributed to physical inactivity, and that a sedentary lifestyle could be among the 10 leading causes of death and disability in the world. Additionally, according to Johns Hopkins Medicine, people who are less active are more likely to develop high blood pressure and coronary heart disease, even in comparison to smokers, while overweight or obese people significantly reduce their risk for disease with regular exercise.

Dr. James A. Levine, M.D, Ph.D. has focused the last three decades on the study of the harm caused by too much sedentariness, and pioneered the science of non-exercise activity thermogenesis (NEAT). He currently serves as a principal investigator for the National Institutes of Health. He has served as an expert to the United Nations, as an invitee to the Presidents Cancer Panel, and as a consultant to governments, internationally. Dr. Levine is also the Dr. Richard F. Emslander Professor of Endocrinology and Nutrition Research, at Mayo Clinic.

In a 2015 article in the publication *Diabetologia*, Dr. Levine explains, *"Sitting too much kills. Epidemiological, physiological, and molecular data suggest that sedentary lifestyle can explain, in part, how modernity is associated with obesity, more than 30 chronic diseases and conditions and high healthcare costs. Excessive sitting-sitting disease is not innate to the human condition. People were designed to be bipedal and, before the industrial revolution, people moved substantially more throughout the day than they do presently."* Per Dr. Levine, excessive sitting is a contributing factor to a legion of chronic illnesses, like type 2 diabetes, cardiovascular disease, and many types of cancer. To maintain your good health and vitality, you *must* move your body every day.

Engaging in physical activity:

» Relieves stress and improves mood

» Raises insulin sensitivity, and helps stabilize blood sugar levels

» Increases the strength and efficiency of the heart and lungs

» Improves circulation

» Strengthens muscles and bones

» Increases flexibility and balance

» Improves sleep

These are all important features of a happy and healthy life. You need strong muscles and bones, as well as a healthy heart and lungs, so you can live a productive, independent, and fulfilled life, and you need good flexibility and balance to get through your everyday activities without injury.

The upside to all this is that the solutions are fairly uncomplicated, once you become aware of the problem. We all have to find ways to keep active daily, and we need to exercise for a minimum of 30 minutes a day, at least 5 days a week. I'll give you a bunch of simple solutions on how to accomplish this painlessly, a little further along in the book.

TOXINS

Our bodies are being constantly exposed to harmful substances. Harmful bacteria, chlorine, lead, and arsenic are commonly found in our tap water. The foods we buy are filled with unhealthy additives, chemicals, pesticides, heavy metals, and preservatives. The air we breathe is filled with car exhaust, smoke, and other pollutants.

It might seem obvious that these toxins and pollutants are harmful to us. What might not be as obvious, is sometimes it only takes an incremental exposure to a toxin for it to have a large impact on our health. Take for example bisphenol A (BPA,) a chemical compound often found in plastics, and Bisphenol S (BPS,) which is now used increasingly as a replacement for BPAs. BPAs are known as endocrine disruptors, and exposure to BPAs have long been linked to cardiovascular disease and obesity. In a recent study, BPS has also been identified as a possible endocrine disruptor. BPS has been linked to the lowering of testosterone and cortisol levels. BPA and BPS have also been linked to the formation of fat, or fatty tissue. These types of toxins are often called obesogens because of their association with weight gain.

Known as "the father of functional medicine," Dr. Jeffrey Bland is a former professor of biochemistry at the University of Puget Sound, and a previous director of nutritional research at the Linus Pauling Institute of Science and Medicine. He's the principal author of over 120 peer-reviewed research papers on nutritional biochemistry. He has authored five books on nutritional medicine for healthcare professionals, and five books on nutrition and health for the general public. In his book

The Disease Delusion, Dr. Bland explains about the harmful effects of bisphenol A. *"It belongs to a large family of chemicals described as endocrine disruptors. The endocrine system is the body's hormonal messaging system, so if it gets disrupted-if messages are altered-the impact on our health can be significant. BPA binds to receptors on cells that the body's natural hormones use to regulate physiological function. In doing so, BPA displaces the natural hormones-basically, knocks them off the receptors and takes their place-and thereby sends different messages to the cells. Moreover, because many of these endocrine-disrupting chemicals are very active, it takes only a very small exposure to create significant changes in health."*

Chemical toxins can affect our endocrine systems and our bodies at a cellular level. Cells are the building blocks of life; they form our organs and contain our DNA. How important to your well-being do you think it is to protect your cells from environmental and dietary toxins? It's for this reason that I use, and advocate the use of, a water filtration system for drinking water, and non-BPA and glass storage containers for food. It's also why I recommend consuming mainly organically grown fruits and vegetables, wild fish; and organic, pastured-raised meat, eggs, dairy, and poultry, as I do.

As we've seen with refined carbohydrates, refined oils, and sugar, sometimes the food itself can be a toxin. There are many people who suffer from food allergies and sensitivities. While not a hazard for everyone, for someone who has a food sensitivity or a food allergy, avoiding specific foods like peanuts, shellfish, or eggs can be a serious matter. These foods are toxic to them, and can make them very ill.

A growing number of people today are experiencing a sensitivity to gluten. Most cases of gluten sensitivity are self-diagnosed, because doctors tend to test for celiac disease (an autoimmune disorder where the ingestion of gluten leads to damage in the small intestine,) and not for gluten sensitivities. The symptoms of a gluten sensitivity are varied, and include bloating, diarrhea, constipation, abdominal pain, headaches, brain fog, and fatigue. (See figure 3 for a list of food items that contain gluten.) Some people also experience a sensitivity to the lactose in dairy products. The symptoms of a lactose sensitivity or intolerance can be very similar to those of someone with a gluten sensitivity.

A common way to test for dietary sensitivities is through an elimination diet. During an elimination diet, the suspect food is removed from the diet for a period of 2-4 weeks. During this time, the person pays careful attention to how they are feeling. If the symptoms ease significantly, or go away completely, the eliminated food may be the cause of discomfort. Some people have reported feeling 100% free of symptoms after being on an elimination diet for only two weeks! If desired, after the prescribed period, the eliminated food can be slowly reintroduced into the diet. If the symptoms return, the person may want to consider permanently removing this food from their diet.

List of Foods That Contain Gluten	
Wheat & wheat germ	Wheat starch
Couscous	Durum
Semolina	Farina
Farro	FV
Gliadin	Graham flour
Kamut	Matzo
Barley	Bulgur
Rye	Seitan
Triticale	Mir
Some veggie burgers	Carmel coloring
Malt	Soy sauce
Some broths	Bran
Some spices	Some dressings
Wheat berries	Brewer's yeast

(Figure 3)

THE MICROBIOME

While discussing things with the power to influence our health and well-being on a cellular level, I cannot leave out the microbiome. The "microbiome" refers to the trillions of microorganisms that live in and on our bodies. Our microbial DNA outnumber, our human DNA by a ratio of 10 to 1. These organisms are key to our health, and we rely on them for our very survival.

A vast amount, roughly 3-5 lbs. of these bacteria, live in our intestines and are called enteric microflora, or gut flora. These gut floras perform many processes that are vital to our existence. They control how efficiently we metabolize our food (if they're too efficient, we get fat; if they're too inefficient, we have trouble keeping weight on and become too thin,) they produce certain vitamins for us, like vitamins k and B12, and they break down complex carbohydrates (like those found in a piece of fruit,) so that we can digest them. The gut microflora also influences our immune responses, and dictates how we respond to foreign invaders and allergens.

There are three classifications of enteric microflora; symbiotic, commensal, and parasitic. The symbiotic bacteria work with our bodies in a way that is mutually beneficial. With the commensal bacteria, the relationship is harmonious, but one sided (they help us, or we help them and neither is harmed.) The parasitic bacteria are of no benefit to us, and they produce substances that can be harmful. Each of these classes of microflora have favorite foods. The good bacteria (symbiotic or commensal) prefer high-fiber plant foods like asparagus, broccoli, cabbage, and raspberries. A diet that is too low in fiber can cause these good bacteria to die, leaving the parasitic bacteria to take their place. The bad or parasitic bacteria love sugar and refined carbohydrates. A diet high in these can lead to an overabundance of these bad bugs, and illness.

Lipopolysaccharide (LPS) is an endotoxin found on the outer membrane of bacterial pathogens. The presence of LPS triggers the release of inflammation causing cytokines, and has been implicated as an early driver of insulin resistance and obesity.

Think of the microbiome as a delicately balanced ecosystem, where diversity and harmony are key. The elimination of one species, or the over population of another, can throw the entire ecosystem out of step, and create havoc on our health. When things are harmonious, it's called symbiosis. When the balance is disturbed, it's known as dysbiosis. Dysbiosis can cause weight gain, inflammation, irritable bowel syndrome, and acid reflux. The influence of the microbiome on our bodies is so massive and far reaching that dysbiosis even effects your brain and mood, causing anxiety, depression, insomnia, and sexual dysfunction.

As reported in a recently published article in *Discovery's Edge*, Mayo Clinic's Research Magazine, *"Practically everything we do-running on a treadmill, popping antibiotics, eating a cheeseburger-shows up in our microbiome. Depending on the environmental input, our gut microbes might turnover completely, or they might churn out chemicals that can predispose us to cancer."*

Dr. Frank Lipman is the founder and director of the Eleven-Eleven Wellness Center in New York City, and a New York Times bestselling author, who has written 4 books. In his online article, "Why Your Microbiome Is Important," he wrote, *"We need the microbiome to keep our gut healthy because the gut is so vital to our overall health. Besides its role in digestion, it also helps us process thought and emotion-so much so that it is often referred to as "the second brain."*

Part of what Dr. Lipman may be referring to is that up to 90% of our serotonin is produced in our gut. Serotonin is a neurotransmitter that influences most of our brain cells. It is believed that serotonin affects mood, bowel function, sexual desire, appetite, sleep, memory, temperature regulation, and blood clotting when there is an injury. In a 2015 study by Caltech, researchers found that up to 60% of the serotonin found in the gut may actually be produced by certain spore-forming species of bacteria.

Most of the intestinal microbiome consists of two bacterial phyla,

Bacteroidetes and Firmicutes. Bacteroidetes are correlated with leanness, while Firmicutes are associated with obesity. Firmicutes become more dominant when we eat a diet that's low in fiber, but high in fat and sugar. Additionally, a 2016 Cornell University study found that dysbiosis, and an abundance of Firmicutes, was a prevalent factor in people suffering from chronic fatigue syndrome.

What we eat not only impacts our own biological functions and hormones, but also has repercussions on the ecological balance of our microbiome. Foods which are probiotic (foods containing beneficial bacteria,) such as yogurt, kefir, and kimchi, promote the growth of a diverse and healthy microbiome. Foods which are prebiotic feed and nourish those good bacteria. (See figure 4 for a list of prebiotic foods)

As per Dr. Gerard E. Mullin, *"Increasing evidence shows that how you feed your gut microbiome is a critical factor in your health and weight."*

Dr. Hyman agrees, *"Food, it turns out, is not just calories but information that radically influences our genes, hormones, immune system, brain chemistry, and even gut flora with every single bite."*

As does Dr. Bland, who wrote, *"A personalized diet program can restore balance to the enteric microflora and change the signals our genes receive."*

Prebiotic Foods List
Apples
Apple cider vinegar
Jerusalem artichokes
Onions
Garlic
Leeks
Dandelion greens
Jicama
Asparagus
Chicory
Under ripe bananas
Canned beans
Cooked and cooled beans
Cashews
Flax seeds
Blueberries
Spinach

(Figure 4)

CHAPTER 4

TIME FOR A CHANGE

LET'S SUM UP WHAT we've covered so far: Processed refined carbohydrates and sugars can cause dysbiosis, chronic inflammation, weight gain, and diseases like diabetes, arterial sclerosis, Alzheimer's, and certain cancers. They have been proven to cause liver damage and cirrhosis. Refined carbohydrates, sugars, and toxins can also trigger negative hormonal and biological reactions within the body.

Certain foods like red meat, alcohol, and gluten can cause inflammation, while other foods like dark chocolate, tart cherries, and ginger are anti-inflammatory. Healthy fats and oils speed up your metabolism, and improve your heart and brain function, all while helping to balance your hormones! High quality carbs provide necessary phytonutrients, vitamins, minerals, and fiber, which prevent cancer, keep us full, and help regulate important body functions, like blood pressure. Additionally, our symbiotic and commensal gut flora love high fiber foods!

Lifestyle and environmental factors like too much stress, too much sitting, and not getting enough sleep are all implicated in chronic problems like weight gain, depression, heart disease, stroke, and insulin resistance, to name just a few. As you can see, there are many complex biological functions that have a huge impact on whether or not we grow fat, or become sick.

The good news is, there is a way out of this dark tunnel! By making manageable changes in lifestyle and nutrition, we can lose weight, improve our health, and change the quality of our lives!

So now let's revisit our original questions: What's going on? Why are so many people overweight? Why are so many people sick?

I've covered most of the biological causes behind our current health dilemmas; now I'd like to address the two biggest health related obstacles we've had to face as a society: I'm talking about the bad advice we've been given for the last 40 years, and our current medical model.

THE MYTH

In the late 1970's the US Senate Select Committee on Nutrition and Human Needs, led by Senator George McGovern, recommended dietary goals for the American people. It was based on an effort to aid in the prevention of chronic diseases, obesity, and heart disease. In 1980, the government put out its very first dietary guidelines for Americans. The guidelines came in the form of a pamphlet full of pertinent information. The pamphlet even contained a height and weight chart, so people would know what their ideal weight should be, and another chart that illustrated how many calories an hour were burned doing different activities. The guidelines where based on the same calories in, calories out theory that we've already discussed, and since fats contain 9 calories per gram, while proteins and carbohydrates contain only 4 calories per gram, people were advised to eat less fat and fatty foods, and to eat more starches and carbohydrates.

Back then, it was believed that foods which contained cholesterol raised blood cholesterol, and since high blood cholesterol was considered a risk factor for heart disease, it made sense to tell people to limit their fat intake. The guidelines became the outline for all future dietary recommendations over the next ten years, and aside from some small alterations, it remained generally the same.

In 1990, suggested serving amounts, and the number of servings recommended, were added to the dietary recommendations. People were instructed to eat 6-11 servings of breads, cereals, pasta, and rice per day. They were encouraged to eat lots of fruit, peas, beans, and starchy vegetables (like potatoes and corn,) on top of those 6-11 servings of cereals and grains. People were also advised to cut their fat intake down to 30% or less of their total daily calories, and to use only vegetable oils in their cooking and on their salads. It was the beginning of the low fat–high carb diet craze.

The combination of lower calories *and* lower cholesterol seemed like a winning concept at the time, but today we know differently. Today we know that it's sugar, and not fat, which raises triglyceride and LDL levels. We also know that having high cholesterol may not be a significant risk factor for cardiovascular disease, and in fact, it may actually prevent it!

In a March 2016 study, researchers studied the official national statistics of food intake against the statistical prevalence of cardiovascular disease. They drew their information from FAOSTAT (the Food and Agricultural Organization of the United Nations Statistical Division,) and from the European cardiovascular disease statistics 2012, which were obtained from World Health Organization databases. The study looked at hundreds of thousands of people, and reviewed data from the years 1965 -2011. The study found that, while eating a high fat, high protein diet does raise blood cholesterol levels, it also lowers the risk for cardiovascular disease. Researchers concluded, after reviewing all the data, that it is carbohydrates and sugars which cause heart disease, and not fat. They cited that low levels of HDL (good cholesterol,) and HDL-cholesterol ratios were the best indicators for the risk of heart disease, and that a high glycemic diet was a key risk factor in getting cardiovascular disease.

I remember a trip to my OBGYN in 1991. I was pregnant with my daughter, and I asked the doctor how I could keep from gaining too much weight during my pregnancy. My doctor advised me to stay away from fat and cholesterol. Seven or eight years later, when I asked my primary care doctor for a weight loss diet, he gave me a copy of the low cholesterol diet, which was basically a breakdown of the same dietary recommended guidelines put out by the government in 1990. (See figure 5 for the exact chart I was given. It might be interesting to note; the chart was created by Parke-Davis, a well-known pharmaceutical company.)

Choose your low-cholesterol, heart-healthy diet

To get the nutrients you need, you have to eat a variety of foods. One way to do this is to choose foods from the different food groups. After determining your dietary goals with your doctor, adjust the number and size of portions to reach and stay at your desired weight.

	Choose	Go Easy	Avoid
Meat, poultry, fish, and shellfish (up to 6 ounces/day)	Lean cuts of meat with fat trimmed, chicken and turkey without skin, fish, shellfish		"Prime"-grade fatty cuts of meat, goose, duck, liver, kidneys, sausage, bacon, regular luncheon meats, hot dogs
Dairy products (2 servings/day; 3 for pregnant or breastfeeding women)	Skim milk, 1% milk, low-fat buttermilk, low-fat evaporated or nonfat milk, low-fat yogurt, cottage cheese, cheeses labeled "no more than 2 to 6 grams of fat per ounce"	2% milk, yogurt, part-skim ricotta, part-skim or imitation hard cheeses (like part-skim mozzarella), "lite" cream cheese, "lite" sour cream	Whole milk, cream, half and half, imitation milk products, whipped cream, custard-style yogurt, whole-milk ricotta, hard cheeses (like Swiss, American, cheddar, muenster), cream cheese, sour cream
Eggs	Egg whites, cholesterol-free egg substitutes	Egg yolks (no more than 3/week)	
Fats and oils (up to 6 to 8 teaspoons/day)	Corn, olive, peanut, canola (rapeseed), safflower, sesame, and soybean oils, tub (not stick) margarine	Nuts, seeds, avocados, olives	Butter, lard, bacon fat, coconut and palm kernel oils
Breads, cereals, pasta, rice, dried peas, and beans (6 to 11 servings/day)	Most breads, bagels, English muffins, rice cakes, low-fat crackers (like matzo, bread sticks, rye krisps, saltines); hot and cold cereals; spaghetti, macaroni, noodles, and any grain rice; dried peas and beans	Store-bought pancakes, waffles, biscuits, muffins, and cornbread	Croissants, sweet rolls, danish, doughnuts, and crackers made with saturated oils; granola-type cereals made with saturated oil, egg noodles, pasta, and rice prepared with cream, butter, or cheese sauce
Fruits and vegetables (2 to 4 servings of fruit/day; 3 to 5 servings of vegetables/day)	Fresh, frozen, canned, or dried fruits		Vegetables prepared in butter, cream, or sauce
Snacks (avoid too many sweets)	Sherbet, sorbet, Italian ice, frozen yogurt, popsicles, angel food cake, fig bars, gingersnaps, low-fat jelly beans and hard candy, plain popcorn, pretzels, fruit juices, tea, coffee	Ice milk, fruit crisps and cobblers, homemade cakes, cookies, and pies prepared with unsaturated oils	Ice cream, frozen tofu, candy, chocolate, potato chips, buttered popcorn, milkshakes, frappes, floats, eggnog, store-bought pies, most store-bought frosted and pound cakes

(P) PARKE-DAVIS   BOOTS PHARMACEUTICALS

A medical service of **PARKE-DAVIS** Division of Warner-Lambert Company, Morris Plains, New Jersey 07950

© 1992 Warner-Lambert Company

(Figure 5)

It was during these years that the food industry, happy to take advantage of the growing new market for low-fat foods, quickly started pumping out all sorts of low-fat products. The problem was that, to have mass appeal, the products had to taste good, and food minus the fat tends to taste a bit like cardboard.

The industry solution to the taste problem was to add more sugar. Thus, we all began eating sugar-filled, low-fat foods, which were produced using the inexpensive and recommended refined vegetable oils. Since high fructose corn syrup is even cheaper than cane sugar, more and more companies began to replace the added sugar in their products with corn syrup. Sweetened cold cereals, fat-free cookies, fat-free ice cream, low-fat granola bars, and sugar-filled low-fat yogurts became the new health foods. Pasta nights were encouraged by health magazines, and by our doctors. Sweetened fruit juices, alcoholic beverages, and candies were even labeled as low-fat health foods! We believed that if a food was low in fat and cholesterol, we could munch away guilt free, and we did. We ate less fat, and consequently less protein. We also ate a lot more carbs, sugar, and calories!

People began eating margarine instead of butter, which was colored with artificial colors, and made more solid by hydrogenating the oils (trans fats). They began cooking with canola and soy bean oil. Coconut oil was vilified. Eggs, avocados, shell fish, nuts, butter, and full-fat dairy products all landed on the list of foods to be avoided.

This giant food myth, and the ensuing food industry trends, quickly spread across most of the developed world. Today, most governmental dietary guidelines closely resemble ours. Since 1980 worldwide obesity has more than doubled, and at least 52% of the world's population is now overweight or obese.

A little bit of knowledge can be a bad thing. Not only did experts at the time *not* understand how to control body weight successfully, but they also made some leaps about the relationship of fat, cholesterol, and heart disease. We unknowingly became the subjects of a huge social experiment. The outcome is a world that is facing an obesity and chronic illness epidemic. Between 1990 and 2010, the total number of deaths caused by cardiovascular diseases increased by more than 25%, and those of chronic kidney disease and diabetes nearly doubled. Ironically, heart disease is now the leading cause of death in the U.S.A.

The dietary guidelines we have all been following since the 1980s were not only incorrect, they were backwards! It's a high fat, low glycemic diet (not a high carb, low fat diet) that prevents obesity, chronic illness, and heart disease. It's the way we used to eat, back when obesity and chronic diseases were not a global epidemic. Sadly, instead of lengthening as they always have in the past, our lifespans are now predicted to be shorter. Despite all of this, very little in our current dietary guidelines has changed.

THE APPROACH

Let's take a look at how the traditional medical model handles patient care.

Have you ever left the doctor's office, prescription in hand, feeling confused, or even a little frustrated? Frustrated, because even though you had asked, you still didn't know why you were experiencing the conditions that spurred you to visit your doctor in the first place? Your doctor might have implied that it was just one of those things that happens at your age, or that it was something you were sadly genetically predisposed to. These types of explanations make the situation seem inevitable, while placing the blame on you for being a certain age, or for having bad genes. Meanwhile, the real dysfunction may not even have been addressed.

Aside from our regular physicals, most of us go to see our doctors when we feel that something is wrong. Regardless of the nature of the problem(s), the doctor has been trained to diagnose your symptoms in an effort to find the right treatment. For this reason, the doctor may order various tests to be done. Once the doctor can put a name on the problem, the proper treatment can be given.

Dr. Siddhartha Mukherjee is an assistant professor of medicine at Columbia University Medical center, and an attending physician at New York Presbyterian/Columbia University Herbert Irving Comprehensive Cancer Center. He is also a Pulitzer Prize winning author for his non-fiction book on cancer, *The Emperor of All Maladies.*

In a 2015 Ted Talk, Dr. Mukherjee said, "*Now, throughout much of the recent history of medicine, we've thought about illness and treatment in terms of a profoundly simple model. In fact, the model is so simple that you could summarize it in six words: have disease, take pill, kill something. Now the reason for the dominance of this model is of course the antibiotic revolution. Many of you might not know this, but we happen to be celebrating the hundredth year of the introduction of antibiotics into the United States.*"

This medical model, started by the antibiotic revolution over one hundred years ago, works extremely well if you are trying to cure an acute, potentially lethal disease, like pneumonia, tuberculosis, or streptococcus. This "name it, pill it, and kill it" model has been so successful in the treatment of acute diseases, that it was a natural transition for doctors to use the same approach in the treatment of chronic diseases.

If your blood pressure is high, you might be put on a beta blocker, which is a drug that blocks the effects of the hormone epinephrine, (also known as adrenaline.) This makes the heart beat more slowly and with less force, thereby reducing your blood pressure. If your blood sugar is high, you might be treated with a drug to mitigate the sugar, or to increase your insulin production. For gastric acid reflux, you would likely be prescribed a proton pump inhibitor (PPI). It works by decreasing the amount of acid produced by the stomach.

The trouble with addressing chronic concerns with the name it, pill it, and kill it approach, is that the *manifestations* of a disease are being treated as if they *are* the disease. In other words, the doctor is often addressing the symptoms, without addressing the root causes. The disease itself inevitably continues to progress. Over time, the symptoms will worsen, while new expressions of the disease will appear. The patient will be given more and more drugs, in response to each new and worsening health concern, yet they will never get well.

This problem is compounded by the fact that most physicians receive less than 20 hours of education on nutrition in medical school, and although most doctors agree that nutrition and lifestyle are important in terms of the treatment and management of chronic disease, only about 32% of them spend any significant time discussing nutrition with patients, and very few refer patients to a dietician or a nutritionist.

There's no denying it, pharmaceuticals have an important role in medicine, and can be very beneficial when used responsibly. However, most drugs prescribed for chronic diseases weren't manufactured for long term consumption, even though that's how they're typically used, and most drugs have serious, even dangerous side effects. In fact, several medications create as many health problems as they treat. For instance, beta blockers (used to lower blood pressure) and statin drugs (used for lowering cholesterol) have both been shown to significantly increase your risk of developing diabetes, and Victoza (an injectable diabetes medication) may potentially cause health issues as serious as thyroid cancer. Aricept (an Alzheimer's medication) may cause seizures and cardiovascular conditions, which can result in an abnormally slow heartbeat.

In the U.S., pharmaceuticals are a huge business. In 2015, Americans spent a jaw dropping estimated net of $310 billion dollars on medicine, up by 8.5% from 2014. Additionally, more than 4 billion prescriptions were dispensed in 2015, with roughly a 10% increase in anti-depressants and anti-diabetes medications, alone. On top of that, big pharma pays doctors to talk about these medications with their patients and with other medical professionals. In 2016, an investigative analysis by the news journal Propublica was jointly published by NPR, the Boston Globe, and the Tampa Bay Times. The analysis showed that doctors who received payments from the medical industry prescribed drugs differently than those who didn't. In fact, the more money doctors received, the more brand-name medications they tended to prescribe, proving that these payments directly correlated with an approach to prescribing that clearly enhanced the drug companies' profits.

Many chronic illnesses can be resolved through diet and lifestyle interventions, but with such big profits at stake, it literally pays to keep you sick, and coming back for more.

In an April 21, 2016 online article, cardiologist Dr. Mark Hyman wrote, "*To think we can treat heart disease by lowering cholesterol, lowering blood pressure and lowering blood sugar with medication is like mopping up the floor while the sink overflows.*"

Additionally, in a May 12, 2016 Facebook post, Dr. David Ludwig wrote, "*Diabetes is by definition a state of carbohydrate intolerance, where the excess builds up as sugar in the blood. The pharmaceutical industry has devised creative ways to deal with this problem, including various types of insulin and drugs that make the body more sensitive to insulin. SGLT inhibitors are a pricey new category of drug that makes the kidneys excrete excess glucose (though with concerning side effects like urinary tract infections and greater risk for diabetic ketoacidosis). How about eating less processed carbohydrate? Then we wouldn't need to convert the kidneys into sugar disposal units.*"

What about prevention? Did you ever wonder how you and yours might avoid the recurrent problems that seem to have taken root in your family tree? Is it really all inescapable?

AN INTRODUCTION TO FUNCTIONAL MEDICINE

Our genes are waiting for the signals from the environment

- Dr. Jeffrey Bland

Type 2 diabetes, hypertension, chronic fatigue, irritable bowel syndrome, allergies, and many other medical problems are all symptoms and manifestations of an underlying dysfunction in the body. Modern medicine treats these symptoms as if they were the dysfunction, and attempts to resolve them with pills. It's time for a change. We need a new perspective on how to deal with chronic diseases, and on prevention.

It's often hard for new ideas to break through years of traditional practice and pervasive thinking. Never the less, 40 years of solid research, carefully conducted scientific studies, and proven findings won't be denied. Today, increasing numbers of doctors are shifting away from the traditional medical model, and are making the move toward functional medicine.

What is functional medicine? Functional medicine, also known as integrative medicine, is the practice of personalized care for the prevention and treatment of chronic diseases.

In conventional medicine, our bodies are routinely viewed as groupings of individual organs such as the heart, the lungs, and the liver. Those organs are cared for by specialized doctors, like cardiologists, pulmonologists, and hepatologists, whose primary focus is within their own medical specialty. The problem is, these organs do not operate independently of one another. The health of one part of the body effects the health of another part, and thus effects our entire body. For example, diabetes often leads to hypertension and cardiovascular disease, which affects blood flow. Impaired blood flow can then lead to a myriad of other issues, including impaired cognitive function, liver disease, and kidney disease.

In functional medicine, the body is viewed as containing seven core physiological processes that interconnect to create a pattern of health. These systems are directly influenced by our genes, our microbiome, and environmental factors such as diet, lifestyle, sleep, environmental toxins, and stress.

Although we are all human, we are not all identical. There are inherent differences in our biological, emotional, and genetic makeups. Some people are more prone to allergies, while others are not. Some are more at risk for developing a specific illness. Some folks need eight or more hours of sleep each night, while others are fine on just six. People react to stress differently. Some have fast metabolisms; some have slow. There are those with strong immune systems, and others with weakened immunity due to illness, surgery, or medication.

These integral differences affect how our bodies react when exposed to various substances and environmental factors, such as the foods we eat and the medications we take. A medication that is beneficial to you could be completely ineffective, or even harmful, when given to someone else. To be truly beneficial, medicine must look at patients as individuals with diverse emotional and biological, needs, strengths, sensitivities, and weaknesses.

This is how functional medicine approaches human health. It recognizes that we are each unique, and thus need individualized care. It's a personalized approach to medicine, geared toward optimal health and wellbeing, which is facilitated by a therapeutic partnership between doctor and patient.

In his book, Dr. Bland explains, *"Grounded in a systems-based understanding of the way the body functions, functional medicine provides the tools we need to change the messages our genes receive so we can shape our own pattern of health. In empowering us to address the chronic illnesses that are the health issue of our time, it is revolutionizing medical practice and changing the face of health care."*

As for the question of prevention, many chronic illnesses, and even cancers, can be prevented by lifestyle and dietary interventions.

In May of 2016, a study done by the Harvard T.H. Chan School of Public Health concluded that almost 50% of all cancers could be prevented by adopting a healthy lifestyle. The healthy lifestyle standards were not smoking, drinking in moderation only, maintaining a healthy BMI, and participating in weekly aerobic activities. Researchers determined, *"A substantial cancer burden may be prevented through lifestyle modification.*

Primary prevention should remain a priority for cancer control."

Dr. Rudolph Tanzi, Ph.D. a pioneer in the field of Alzheimer's research (having co-discovered the three genes that cause early-onset familial Alzheimer's disease,) is a Professor of Neurology, and the holder of the Joseph P. and Rose Kennedy Endowed Chair in Neurology at Harvard University. He also serves as vice-chair of neurology, and is the director of the Genetics and Aging Research Unit at Massachusetts General Hospital.

Dr. Deepak Chopra, M.D., F.A.C.P., is a respected leader in the field of integrative medicine. He is the founder of the Chopra Foundation, and a co-founder of the Chopra Center for well-being. He serves as adjunct Professor at two well respected universities, and is the assistant clinical professor in the Family and Preventative Medicine Department at the University of California in San Diego.

In their book, *Super Genes*, Dr. Tanzi and Dr. Chopra wrote, *"The news everyone should hear is that Gene activity is largely under our control."* They then go on to say, *"The most exciting news of all is that the conversation between body, mind and genes can be transformed. This transformation goes far beyond prevention, even beyond wellness, to a state we call radical well-being."*

Each of us deserves to unlock the gateway to our own radical well-being.

CHAPTER 5

HEALTHY BODY CONNECTION, THE ANSWER

WITH SO MANY PEOPLE suffering from obesity, heart disease, type 2 diabetes, autoimmune diseases, and other chronic illnesses, the situation appears to be bleak, but there is a silver lining. Our futures don't have to be so grim. We can easily make the necessary changes to live longer, healthier, and better lives. We have the power to reduce our risks for disease, and to create our own good health.

You and your family are not genetically doomed to be sick with the diseases that may have plagued the generations before you. Even if you've been unfortunate enough to have already developed a chronic illness, you can take steps to improve your health and your quality of life. With some straightforward dietary and lifestyle changes, you have a chance to slow, and even reverse, the progression of illness!

You have the power. You can start making a difference in your own life, and in the lives of your family today! All you need is the information.

I have spent years gathering and sorting through the facts and the science. I have done this for myself, my future clients, and for you. I have sifted through and systemized the data, and I've put it all into one simple, easy-to-follow plan, which I call the *Healthy Body Connection Plan*.

The great scientific minds of today, whose work I have studied (scientists, researchers, doctors, and experts alike,) all clearly agree on certain fundamental aspects of diet, lifestyle, and the direct relationship it has on our health and longevity. These fundamentals are the core principles of the *Healthy Body Connection Plan.*

Since functional medicine recognizes that individual lifestyles, genotypes, and environmental factors all influence our respective health patterns, I have come to realize that many of the discrepancies (the things the experts don't seem to be able to agree on) are based more on individuality, than on hard and fast rules. There is no cookie cutter, "one size fits all" approach that will work for everyone. We are all unique; we each have different health needs, and genetic strengths and predispositions. As such, we need to learn what works best for ourselves as individuals.

In the following pages, I'll map out the core principles of the *Healthy Body Connection Plan.* I'll explain how you can use these core principles to personalize your own diet and lifestyle plan. I'll do my best to lay everything out in a clear and simple manner. I hope you'll take the information and run with it. I want you to feel inspired to know that you can live your best life. I want you to feel empowered to know that you can achieve not only weight loss, but, more importantly, optimal health and wellbeing.

It's all possible, but first you must be willing to let go of some of the old notions that have been drummed into your head. You'll have to let go of habits like restricting your calories. You'll have to learn to listen to your body, and to pay attention to hunger and satiety cues. It can be difficult, and even a little scary at times, but believe me when I tell you that your body is amazing! You'll get the best results when you learn how to work with your body, instead of against it. Next, you must be willing to make a commitment to yourself, and to making some changes in your diet and lifestyle. It might seem a little daunting at first, but it really isn't that hard, and you'll be glad you made the effort.

To help you begin, I'll cover the important dietary components of the plan. I'll answer all your questions about what foods to eat, and what foods to avoid. I promise you that you'll never feel deprived. You can even eat cupcakes and breads, if they're made with the right ingredients! You'll find a variety of delicious recipes for items like these (and many others,) right in the recipe section of this book. The recipes are so good; before you know it, the whole family will be eating better, and feeling healthier.

On the *Healthy Body Connection Plan*, you'll be eating rich, satisfying, delicious meals. The best part is that you'll never be asked to go hungry, or to leave the table wanting more, and you'll never have to count calories again! Following your body's natural hunger cues, or mindful eating, is a key component of this plan. You'll learn exactly how to combine mindful eating with healthy eating, and how to personalize your dietary intake to help you achieve the best results. I'll also lightly cover the topic of vitamins, minerals, and other supplements that you may want to consider asking your doctor about.

After that, we'll move on to some lifestyle strategies. Before you know it, you'll not only feel better; you'll be sleeping better, you'll have lots more energy, and you'll have drastically improved the quality of your health and your life!

I'm so excited, because I know that each of you can fulfill your potential to live a longer, better, and happier life! So, what are we waiting for? Let's get started!

AN OVERVIEW

Our good health is our first wealth. Without good health, nothing else matters. Life can't be fully enjoyed when we're sick and feeling lousy. That being said, I have done my best to create the healthiest possible dietary and lifestyle plan.

Please be aware that the *Healthy Body Connection Plan* will likely lower your blood sugar levels, your blood pressure, and may even help

balance your hormone levels. Please fully consult with your doctor before starting the *Healthy Body Connection plan*. Additionally, if you have any medical conditions, are taking any medications, or are being treated with hormone replacement therapy and you begin the *Healthy Body Connection Plan*, you will need careful, continuous monitoring by your doctor, so that they can adjust and/or lower your prescriptions as necessary.

The *Healthy Body Connection Plan* is a three-stage plan. The Healthy Start is where all the prep-work begins. During this stage, you'll get yourself and your home ready for the changes that are about to come.

The Able Body stage is next. This stage is a time for detoxifying, healing, and being kind to yourself. The Able Body stage prepares your body, and sets you up for sustainable weight loss and good health.

The Daily Connection stage comes next. In this stage, you'll be paying close attention to certain foods and how they affect you. You'll continue to lose weight, and you should begin to feel better, too. You'll notice that you're having fewer cravings, less hunger, and more energy. During this stage, you'll also be adding in some positive lifestyle changes, to help you on your way to a healthier body and a better, happier life!

WHAT YOU'LL BE EATING AND DRINKING

Organic, Wild, and Pasture Raised Foods

On the *Healthy Body Connection Plan*, you'll be consuming real, whole foods, consisting mainly of organically grown fresh fruits and vegetables, wild fish, and grass-fed lamb, chicken, and beef. You can also choose to eat wild game, like bison, elk, and venison, if you like. Your dairy and eggs should also be organic, and come from pasture-raised animals.

Organically grown fruits and vegetables are free of many of the harmful pesticides and chemicals that are present in non-organic produce. Organic foods taste much better, too. In fact, when I first began eating organically grown foods, I was blown away by the noticeable increase in sweetness, flavor, and quality!

Pasture raised and wild meats contain higher levels of healthy omega 3 fats, and are a better source of nutrition than their grain fed counterparts. Non-organic, corn- and grain-fed meats, dairy products, and eggs are all full of hormones, antibiotics, and pesticides. Corn-fed meats also contain more inflammatory omega 6 fats, and fewer anti-inflammatory omega 3 fats.

Wild fish, like Alaskan salmon, herring, and sardines, are all high in beneficial omega 3 fats. Other healthy choices include anchovies, clams, haddock, flounder, crab, and wild American shrimp. These types of fish are low in mercury, and may safely be eaten 2-3 times a week. Canned light tuna, halibut, cod, snapper, and lobster contain a moderate amount of mercury, and consumption should be limited to about once a week. Fish like bluefish, mackerel, Chilean sea bass, swordfish, canned albacore tuna, ahi tuna, tile fish, and orange roughy should all be avoided, due to the high mercury levels commonly found in these fish. Farm-raised fish should also be avoided, because they are full of pollutants, pesticides, and harmful chemicals. Additionally, farm raised fish have been found to be less nutritious, and they contain fewer omega 3s than the wild caught varieties.

I know that buying organic, wild, and pasture-raised foods can be more expensive than buying non-organic foods, but to me, the benefits are well worth the extra expense. Plus, you'll be saving money on all the junk that you'll no longer be buying.

Initially, it can be easy to overspend at the grocery store. Over time, you'll gain a better sense of how much food you really need to purchase each week. Plus, after the first week or two, you'll have a well-stocked pantry, and you'll only have to replace things as you use them. At that point, you should see your grocery bills begin to return to normal.

Truthfully, though, wouldn't you rather choose to spend a little extra money on delicious, healthy foods than be forced to spend a lot of extra money on expensive medications and trips to the doctor's office, (or even worse, to the hospital?)

A Rainbow of Fruits and Vegetables

Fresh fruits and vegetables come in every color of the rainbow. For optimal nutrition, we need to eat the full spectrum of colors, from plant based foods, every day. The best way to do this is to include 3 - 4 servings of different fruits and/or vegetables at each meal, because we need 9-12 servings daily. A serving size is roughly ½ cup of raw or cooked vegetables, 1 cup of raw leafy greens, 1 cup of berries, ½ cup of cut fruit, or 1 medium-sized piece of whole . (See the Rainbow Food Chart below, in figure 6).

You can eat your daily 9-12 servings separately, or you can combine 3 or 4 at a time to create exciting, healthful main courses and side dishes. For example, you could add some sautéed asparagus and onions with fresh tomato slices to your morning omelet, or you could make a fresh salad for lunch with ingredients like fresh spinach, walnuts, apple chunks, and carrot slices. You could add a variety of fresh berries and pumpkin seeds to your yogurt, or make colorful stir-fries for side dishes or main meals. The options are endless, and besides the valuable phytonutrients that you'll be adding to each meal, you'll also be adding great flavor. Any good chef will tell you that the more colorful a meal is, the better it usually tastes!

Some foods, when eaten in combination, boost each other's nutritional value or nutritional availability. Combining iron rich foods with vitamin C rich foods can help your body to absorb the iron better. So, squeezing some lemon juice onto your cooked greens or seafood is a smart choice. The same thing happens when you combine lycopene (found in tomatoes, red grapefruit, and watermelon,) with fats; it increases the absorption of lycopene. Sulforaphane (which is found in foods like broccoli, Brussels sprouts, and cauliflower,) combined with selenium (found in nuts, eggs, and mushrooms) can help to fight cancer. Getting creative can be fun, too. By trying different combinations, you can create your own personal masterpieces!

RED FOODS		
Apples	Cranberries	Pomegranates
Beans (Adzuki, Red, Red Kidney)	Cherries	Radicchio
Beets	Pink or Red Grapefruit	Radishes
Red Peppers	Red Grapes	Raspberries
Blood Oranges	Red Onions	Strawberries
Tomatoes	Watermelon	Red Plums
Red Pears		
ORANGE FOODS		
Oranges	Nectarines	Papaya
Tangerines	Peaches	Sweet Potatoes and Yams
Cantaloupe	Apricots	Winter Squash (Butternut, Acorn)
Orange Bell Peppers	Pumpkin	Mangos
YELLOW FOODS		
Golden Delicious Apples	Bananas	Star Fruit
Lemons	Corn	Grapefruit
Asian Pears	Pineapple	Summer Squash
Yellow Pears	Yellow Watermelon	Yellow Tomatoes
Yellow Beets	Yellow Carrots	Spagetti Squash
GREEN FOODS		
Green Apples	Honeydew	Asparagus
Green Pears	Kiwi Fruit	Green Beans
Green Grapes	Avacado	Brussels Sprouts
Limes	Artichokes	Broccoli
Broccolini	Bell Peppers	Celery
Cabbage	Bok Choy	Cucumbers
Peas	Leafy Greens (Arugula, Beet Greens	Okra
Snow Peas	Kale, Spinach, Dandilion, etc.)	Zucchini
Green Onions & Leeks	Snow Peas & Sugar Snap Peas	
PURPLE/BLUE FOODS		
Blackberries	Eggplant	
Blueberries	Purple/Black Grapes	
Boysenberries	Purple/Black Plums	
Purple Cabbage	Figs	
Purple Carrots	Prunes & Raisins	
Purple Potatoes	Purple Kale	
WHITE/TAN/BROWN FOODS		
Brown Pears	Onions	Mushrooms
Dates	Parsnips	Beans
Lychee Fruit	White Carrots	Nuts
Cauliflower	Garlic	Shallots
Sauerkraut	Seeds	Whole Grains
Raw Cacao	Cocoa	Coconut
Ginger	White Nectarines & Peaches	Turnips

(Figure 6 - Rainbow Food Chart)

Fresh Herbs and Spices

The right combination of fresh (or even dried) herbs & spices can transform a dish from the mundane to the sublime. The right mixture can give food a unique flavor profile or a distinct ethnic flare, but, more importantly, herbs and spices also possess many unique health-promoting properties.

Throughout history, many different cultures have used herbs and spices for medicinal purposes. They can be anti-inflammatory, antimicrobial, and anti-fungal. They can help lower blood pressure, promote liver health, ease nausea, and much more. Herbs & spices can also be useful in managing and reducing the risks for chronic diseases, like diabetes and heart disease.

Let's talk about a few more commonly found herbs & spices, and their healthy properties.

» Cinnamon helps lower blood sugar levels and LDL (bad cholesterol). It also increases insulin sensitivity, which helps burn fat and calories.

» Ginger is known for its digestive properties. It helps reduce nausea, and it's anti-inflammatory as well.

» Turmeric and cumin have strong anti-inflammatory properties, and have been linked to the detoxification and protection of the liver, as well as reducing the risk for skin cancer.

» Oregano has as many antioxidants as 3 whole cups of broccoli, in just one tsp. It's also good for digestion, and respiratory health.

» Rosemary is another anti-inflammatory herb. Reducing inflammation in the body is vital to heart health and brain function. Inflammation has also been shown to be a precursor to diabetes.

» Thyme is known to stimulate the immune system.

» Cayenne is linked to increased metabolism, which is great for weight control. Cayenne is also associated with the easing of cold and flu symptoms.

» Sage, when brewed as a tea, is often used to sooth a sore throat, and to help reduce excessive sweating.

» Parsley can reduce the risk for certain cancers, and helps inhibit atherosclerosis (hardening of the arteries.)

» Garlic, onions, and leeks help to lower LDL cholesterol levels, and have anti-cancer properties.

» Black pepper contains a naturally occurring compound called piperine. Piperine helps the body better absorb many vitamins, minerals, and nutrients from food. For example, the curcumin in turmeric cannot be well-absorbed on its own, but when paired with piperine, bioavailability improves drastically.

Try to incorporate herbs and spices into your meals whenever possible. You can use dried herbs and spices for convenience, but the fresh variety tastes better and are more potent. To save money, you can grow many fresh herbs in your garden. If you're short on outdoor space, you can grow them in small pots on your patio, or on a sunny window sill, for a wonderful little herb garden, indoors!

Full Fat Dairy Products

Butter and dairy products have been a source of controversy and confusion for years. If you're going to eat dairy and butter spreads, it's best to stick with real butter and full fat dairy, from organic, grass fed cows. Butter is far superior to margarine, (which is often made with highly processed oils and artificial ingredients,) and low-fat dairy products have more lactose sugar. Full fat dairy is also more satisfying, and will keep you full for longer. Dairy products are a good source of calcium, vitamin D, and protein. In particular, full fat plain Greek yogurt is higher in protein than regular yogurt, and is also a source of health-promoting probiotics.

That being said, you still might want to go easy when it comes to dairy. Studies have shown that, although dairy products have a relatively low glycemic index, they produce high insulin responses in the body. Hyperinsulinemia (too much insulin in the blood) is one of the symptoms of pre-diabetes, which leads to insulin resistance and diabetes. It's not clear what it is about milk that causes this high insulin response, but some think it could be due to the whey proteins which are found in milk.

In a 2009 Denmark study, researchers studied 57 eight-year-old boys to determine which components in milk are responsible for its growth-stimulating effect. They found that the proteins in milk (casein and whey,) and not the minerals, were responsible for the growth-promoting effect. More interestingly, they also found that whey protein increased the boys' fasting insulin response, while the casein did not.

Some dairy products which contain the most whey are: milk, cream, yogurt, sour cream, cottage cheese, and ricotta. If you have a strong family history of type 2 diabetes, have been told by your doctor that you are pre-diabetic, insulin resistant, or if you already have type 2 diabetes, limit your consumption of these foods, and avoid whey protein powders and whey protein shakes.

Whey is usually disposed of as a waste product in the cheese-making process, so cheeses such as cheddar, gouda, Swiss, and cream cheese seem to cause a much lower insulin response in comparison to other milk products. While these do seem like better choices, my advice remains the same. Go easy on the dairy. A little cream in your coffee probably won't kill you, and a piece of cheese now and then is lovely, but consider that there are healthier fats available to you. Save dairy products for an occasional snack or treat.

Whole Eggs

Due to a fear of eating fat, high cholesterol, and extra calories, for years we've been advised to choose egg whites over whole eggs. We now know that fat is not to be feared, and that dietary cholesterol has little to do with the cholesterol in our blood.

Whole eggs are delicious, and full of nutrition. Most of the nutrition found in an egg comes from the yolk. One whole egg has 7 grams of protein, as well as iron, vitamins, minerals, and carotenoids. Carotenoids are responsible for the egg yolks sunny yellow color, and may reduce the risk of age-related macular degeneration, the leading cause of blindness in older adults.

Whole eggs also contain an essential nutrient called choline. Choline is necessary for many physiological processes. Brain development and memory may be enhanced by the choline content of eggs. A choline deficiency can cause muscle damage, and abnormal deposits of fat in the liver, resulting in a condition called nonalcoholic fatty liver disease. So, in conclusion: Whole eggs are in, and (for the most part) egg whites are out!

Healthy Fats and Omega 3s

Healthy fats, like avocado, nuts, seeds, coconut, coconut oil, olives, and olive oil, will be included at every meal, and even at snack time. These good fats promote healthy skin, hair, and nails. They're anti-inflammatory, and they help support vascular, heart, and brain health. Remember, also, that fats are more readily used for energy, and are less likely to be stored as fat in the body, because dietary fats have little to no effect on insulin secretion, and without insulin there is no fat storage.

Dark Chocolate

Flavonoid-rich foods like dark chocolate, red wine, and tea are believed to decrease the risk of death from coronary heart disease, cancer, and stroke. Additionally, the consumption of dark chocolate has been shown to improve vascular health, decrease blood pressure, and decrease insulin resistance. However, due to the added sugar, eating large quantities of dark chocolate may be too much of a good thing. Therefore, enjoying 1 oz. of dark chocolate (70% cacao or more) daily, is encouraged.

Water

50% - 70% of our body is composed of water, and the human body can only go for a handful of days without water. Water is used for many vital biological functions, like maintaining blood pressure, lubricating joints, and regulating core body temperature. To stay hydrated, you should drink plenty of filtered water throughout the day. The average person needs approximately one half their body weight in ounces of water, daily. So, for example, if you weigh 160 lbs., you need to drink 80 oz. of water (or about 10 glasses) spread out over the course of each day. It's important to make sure your water is filtered, and safe from dangerous chemicals, toxins, and pollutants. There are many good water filtering systems available, both online and in your local hardware store. You can purchase a complete under-the- counter water filtration kit, for your kitchen sink, for about one hundred dollars. It's a pretty cost-effective way to ensure that you always have safe water for cooking and drinking.

Coffee & Tea

After water, coffee and tea are the two most commonly enjoyed beverages in the world.

There have been multiple studies conducted as to the many health benefits of drinking coffee. Coffee contains vitamin B2, and many phytochemical antioxidants. In fact, coffee is the largest source of phytochemicals in the American diet. Since the roasting process burns off some of these phytochemicals, light to medium roasts contain more beneficial antioxidants than dark roasts, which have been roasted longer. Researchers have found that coffee consumption is associated with a decreased risk for multiple sclerosis, type 2 diabetes, and certain cancers. The American Institute for Cancer Research even has coffee on its list *AICR's Foods That Fight Cancer.*

Tea is well-regarded for its health-promoting catechins. Catechins are phytochemical compounds, found in high concentrations in a variety of plant-based foods and beverages, such as tea, dark chocolate, and blackberries. Consumption of catechins has been linked with a variety of beneficial effects including increased plasma antioxidant activity and weight loss. Black tea and green tea have both been associated with lowering LDL cholesterol, improving blood flow, reducing blood pressure, and preventing cancer.

Although most of us can't imagine getting through the morning without the caffeine boost from our morning cup of coffee or tea, too much caffeine can be problematic. Everyone's tolerance level is different, but consuming too much caffeine can lead to acid reflux, palpitations, dehydration, feelings of anxiety or nervousness, and difficulty sleeping at night. Some experts advise that consuming too much caffeine can also cause a decrease in insulin sensitivity.

Depending on your personal tolerance level, it's advisable to limit your consumption of caffeinated beverages to 2-3 cups per day. Decaffeinated tea or coffee may be enjoyed in unlimited amounts. When purchasing decaffeinated coffee, it's a good idea to buy organic coffee. Organic coffees are decaffeinated with water, and without the use of harmful chemicals.

Wine/Alcoholic Beverages

The good news is that alcoholic beverages, especially red wine, *are* on-plan in *moderation*. Red wine contains beneficial phytochemicals, such as resveratrol. Like dark chocolate, coffee, and tea, red wine has been associated with many health-protecting benefits, when consumed in moderation.

In keeping with the CDC, drinking in moderation equates to 1 drink per day for women, and 2 drinks per day for men. A drink is defined as 12-ounces of beer, 8-ounces of malt liquor, 5-ounces of wine, or 1.5-ounces of liquor.

Drinking too much alcohol is dangerous to the health of your brain, your liver, and your microbiome. While alcoholic beverages are permitted on the HBC plan, some of you may find that alcohol consumption interferes with your weight loss/health goals, and may need to abstain from drinking alcoholic beverages for a time.

WHAT YOU WON'T BE EATING

Refined Carbohydrates & Processed Food

Usually made with unhealthy preservatives, manmade chemical additives, artificial flavors, and artificial colors, some processed, packaged foods shouldn't even be considered food! On top of that, they're loaded down with sugar, high fructose corn syrup, salt, and inexpensive unhealthy oils.

As you've probably guessed by now, there will be a minimal amount of sugar, and absolutely no refined carbohydrates or processed foods on this plan. Refined carbohydrates are any carbohydrate foods that have been processed in a way that speeds up how quickly they're digested. So, for example, a fresh apple is an unrefined, whole food. Applesauce, however, is refined, because it has been cooked down, and condensed. It will be digested faster than a fresh apple, and it will cause your blood sugar to spike.

All flours made from grains (even whole grains) are refined carbohydrates. Traditionally baked products made from these flours are refined carbohydrates, too. Foods like bread, bread crumbs, cakes, pies, crackers, pretzels, and cookies all fall into this category. These foods, along with processed packaged foods, like packaged ice cream, frozen and boxed dinners, chips, candies, and sugary drinks, are all off-plan.

On the *Healthy Body Connection Plan*, you'll still be able enjoy breads, rolls, and even yummy desserts, they'll just be made with different ingredients. Additionally, you'll always be in control, and you'll know exactly what's in the food you're eating, because you'll be preparing most of it yourself. You'll be enjoying things like cupcakes, breads, casseroles, pancakes, desserts, great meals, snacks, and dips! Quick and easy recipes, for these items and more, can be found in the recipe section of this book, along with some meal ideas and helpful tips. Even if you've never cooked before, you'll be able to follow these simple recipes. What's more, all the recipes are nutritious, grain-free, low in sugar, and (most importantly) delicious. There's even a great recipe for a pizza!

What About Artificial Sweeteners?

You might think that artificial sweeteners or other "natural sweeteners" like stevia are alright, but I disagree. Artificial sweeteners are super sweet, making everything else taste like they aren't sweet enough, by comparison, including healthy fruits and vegetables. Because they taste so sweet, they can trick our brains and trigger an insulin response. Additionally, the over-sweetness of artificial sweeteners causes sugar cravings. They can also be addictive, and they're full of chemicals that our bodies weren't meant to process.

Tim Spector is a professor of Genetic Epidemiology, and is the director of the TwinsUK Registry at Kings College, London, and has recently been elected to the prestigious Fellowship of the Academy of Medical Sciences. In a 2015 online article, published by The Spectator, Dr. Spector wrote these words regarding the effect that different food substances have on our microbiome, "*When our microbes are disrupted it makes us sick. It turns out that our microbes dislike these 'harmless' substances like emulsifiers, preservatives, and artificial sweeteners, making them produce unusual obesity- and diabetes-promoting chemicals and killing off many friendly species. Microbes in our mouth can also convert nitrites to nitrosamines – a classic carcinogen.*"

To sum things up, artificial sweeteners are substances which make us fat, and increase our risk for diabetes.

Stevia is no better, because it requires processing to make it palatable. There is insufficient data on how safe it really is, and the FDA has not approved it for use as a food additive. Although stevia is considered a natural substance, just because it's natural doesn't mean it's healthy. Remember: arsenic is natural, too. I choose to err on the side of caution, so for this reason, stevia is also not on-plan.

Trans Fats and Refined Vegetable Oils

Vegetable oils like soy, corn, canola, cotton seed, sunflower, and safflower are all refined oils. Refined oils have been treated with high temperatures and caustic chemicals, which make them an unhealthy option. Refined vegetable oils are also high in inflammatory omega 6 fats. Too many omega 6 fats in our diets, in combination with too few omega 3 fats, promotes the pathogenesis of many diseases including cardiovascular disease, cancer, inflammatory diseases, and autoimmune diseases. So, be sure to avoid these oils, and any foods prepared with or containing them.

Soy Products

For some, soy consumption can be a very controversial topic.

Soy, long regarded as a great source of vegetable protein, contains phytoestrogens. A phytoestrogen is a plant estrogen that exerts an estrogen-like action on the body. For years, tofu (which is made from soy) was considered a health food, and many vegetarians still eat tofu and other soy products as a replacement for meat-based protein. However, due to its estrogen-like effects on the body, eating too much is not a good idea. As I stated earlier, too much estrogen can have an adverse effect on your health. Eating soy may interfere with hormonal balance, and throw off your body's natural processes. There is also a concern that consuming soy-based phytoestrogens may be linked to an increased risk for breast cancer in adults, and for infants who are fed soy formula.

Studies done on the pros and cons of soy consumption have had consistently opposing findings. While some studies have found soy consumption to be beneficial to our health, other studies have shown soy consumption to be linked to a higher risk for breast cancer, and for reproductive issues in both men and women. According to a paper published in the journal Front Neuroendocrinol in 2010, the benefits of soy consumption varied largely by the race and age of the subjects studied. Authors Heather Patisaul, Ph.D., an Assistant Professor at North Carolina State University, and Wendy Jefferson, Ph.D., a biologist, concluded that, "*While the potentially beneficial effects of phytoestrogen consumption have been eagerly pursued, and frequently overstated, the*

potentially adverse effects of these compounds are likely underappreciated."
They recommended, *"Consumers should be aware that soy contains endocrine disrupting compounds and make dietary choices accordingly."* Remember, the endocrine system is the body's hormonal messaging system. Anything that disrupts that system can have a significant impact on our health. The scientists also warned, *"Women who are pregnant, nursing or attempting to become pregnant should use soy foods with caution and be aware that soy formula may not be the best option for their babies."*

I personally don't eat soy products, and I don't recommend them. If you choose to use soy products, do so cautiously and limit your intake to no more than once or twice a week. Men with low testosterone levels should not eat soy products, at all.

AN INTRODUCTION TO MINDFUL EATING

Over the years, most of us have believed that the only way to lose weight was by restricting our calories and our food intake. Now we understand that what you eat is so much more important than how much you eat, because the calorie in calorie out line of thinking doesn't account for how food is metabolized by our bodies, or by our enteric microflora. You already know that dieting and calorie restriction just doesn't work, because we can't fight our own biology. The body is self-regulating, and that's where the magic lies!

If you listen to your body and the cues it gives you, you can never go wrong. Your body will tell you how much to eat, and when to eat. When you make the right food choices, and listen to the cues your body is sending you, you will begin to gain better health, while your body returns to its natural weight set point. For most people who are overweight, this will equate to sustainable weight loss over time.

So, how do you accomplish this? It's simple. You eat nourishing, satisfying meals, in accordance with the nutritional information given in *The Healthy Body Connection Plan,* and you follow a few, straightforward guidelines, as follows:

1. **Eat when you're hungry,** and only when you're hungry. Never eat a meal just because it's noon, or six pm.

2. **Eat slowly.** Take the time to chew your food, and to enjoy your meal. When you eat too quickly, it's harder to notice when you're full, and it's easy to eat more than you need.

3. **Take a reasonable portion size.** You can always take more, if you're still hungry after it's gone. It's easy to overeat if you start out with too much in your plate.

4. **Stop eating when you feel full**, but not over-stuffed. You should feel satisfied, comfortable, and no longer hungry when you're done eating, but you shouldn't feel so full that you don't want to move, like after a big holiday feast. A good rule of thumb is to stop eating when you feel 80-90% full.

5. **Wait** 15-20 minutes before going back for seconds. Sometimes it takes a while for your brain to catch up with your stomach, and tell you that you're full.

6. **Never leave the table hungry**. If you find that you are still hungry, go get more food! Try going back for more veggies, a little more protein, or both.

7. **Eat whenever you feel *physically* hungry**. There are no rules on how many meals a day you can or must eat. If you're hungry between meals, by all means, have a snack! Just make sure you are eating because you feel physically hungry, and not because of other reasons like boredom, emotional distress, or to be social.

8. **If you're not hungry, don't eat**. You may find that after a good breakfast, you're not hungry for hours! Again, eat in accordance with your own body. If breakfast was at 8am but you're not hungry until 3pm, don't eat again until 3pm.

At first it may be difficult to *hear* what your body is saying. It takes a little time and attention, but over time it, will get easier. You may also find it hard to stop worrying about how many calories you're eating, but have faith in the fact that the body is amazing and knows exactly how much it needs. Your body will adjust your caloric intake from one day to the next, based on your activity levels, how much rest you're getting, and your physical needs. You're going to be astonished by how much better you are eating. You'll find that you're eating more food than before, and still losing weight!

So, forget about counting calories. Life is too short to spend so much time obsessing over meaningless numbers! Just feed your body the nourishing foods that it needs, and listen to the messages that your body is sending you. The rest will take care of itself.

CHAPTER 6

THE PLAN

STAGE ONE – THE HEALTHY START

Any great endeavor takes a bit of preparation. To prepare for this exciting new chapter in your life, you'll need to do a few things.

1. Make an appointment

Make an appointment with your physician for a full physical exam. While you're there, discuss any health concerns that you have with your doctor, and explain your intentions of starting the Healthy Body Connection Plan. Make sure that he/she is fully aware of the plan details (you may even want to bring a copy of the book with you for your doctor to look at,) and get your doctor's approval to begin. To give you a starting baseline, I would recommend having your doctor run a few basic blood tests such as:

>> *a fasting insulin test – too much insulin in the blood could signal insulin resistance or pre-diabetes*
>> *a hemoglobin A1C - to check your blood glucose levels*
>> *a lipid profile - to check your cholesterol levels*
>> *a THS - to check your thyroid function.*

This would also be a great time to have your doctor check for vitamin and mineral deficiencies, or any other possible hormonal imbalances.

2. Rally your support

Tell the people who mean the most to you of your intentions to start the Healthy Body Connection Plan. Involving others who care about you will give you accountability and a support network to help make things easier. Ask them for their support. Tell them what it will mean to you and how it will impact your future. Let them know how much you appreciate their continued support, encouragement, positivity, and help. Maybe you can even find someone to do the plan with. Having a partner to share your adventure with makes the whole experience a lot more fun!

3. Out with the old

Time to clear your pantry shelves, your refrigerator, and your freezer of all the old refined carbs, processed foods, sugar, and junk. Get rid of the sugar filled jams and jellies, ketchups, BBQ sauces, candies, breads, cereals, pretzels, chips, frozen pizzas, and packaged dinners. Throw out the pasta, the rice, and the rolled oats. Toss away the hot dogs and processed meats, the low-fat yogurt, and the skim milk. Make room for all the fresh, wonderful foods that are about to become a part of your new, better life!

4. In with the new

Now you can make a shopping list based on the approved Able Body Foods List (pages 94-101), and start restocking your home with delicious things, like fresh fruits and vegetables; grass-fed lamb, chicken, & beef; wild Alaskan salmon and shellfish; olive oil, coconut oil, coconut milk; walnuts, almonds, and cashews; pastured, fresh eggs; grass-fed butter, and don't forget the dark chocolate!

STAGE TWO – THE ABLE BODY

The Able Body Stage is a 2-week detoxification period that primes your body, and gets you ready for success. Think of it like turning to a new page in your personal book of life. On a clean page, you can begin to write a new chapter that begins your own story of health and wellness.

For just these two weeks, there will be no grains, no sugar, no potatoes, no starchy vegetables, no high glycemic tropical fruits, no dried fruits, and no alcohol. Don't worry though, there will be plenty of food, including low glycemic fruits and vegetables, proteins, and healthy fats to eat.

During this stage, your body will be going through a process that is very similar to withdrawal. While many people will get through this phase without incident, to be fair, I'll tell you that there will be some who may not feel very well during this adjustment period. There is the possibility that you may feel lethargic, or more tired than usual. You may even get headaches, or feel queasy.

Drinking lots of water and making sure to get enough rest will help. If your doctor allows, try adding a little iodized sea salt to your diet each day. It will help you stay hydrated, and help prevent constipation. If you experience constipation, a magnesium supplement may help (see the Supplement Page for more detailed info,) and so will adding a tablespoon of ground flax seeds to one or more meals per day.

Also, this would not be the time to start any new strenuous exercise programs. These two weeks are a time to reset and relax. If you already participate in regular physical activities, go a little easy during this stage.

I recommend that you also remove dairy, and extend this stage to 3 weeks, if you have been diagnosed with an autoimmune disease, or if you suffer from any of the following: skin rashes, eczema, brain fog, chronic fatigue, unexplained joint or muscle pains, headaches, bloating, excessive gas, constipation, diarrhea, or other digestive issues. By doing this, it will be easier to pinpoint possible food sensitivities later on in stage 3, which might be contributing to, aggravating, or possibly even causing these issues.

Hang in there. Two or three weeks is only a drop in the bucket. I know you can do it, and I promise it'll be well worth it. Soon, your energy levels will be soaring, and you'll be feeling better than ever!

SOME KEY POINTERS BEFORE YOU START

These apply to both stages 2 & 3

» Start every day with a large glass of filtered water. This will rehydrate you and wake your system up. Make sure to stay properly hydrated by drinking plenty of water throughout the day, too.

» Eating seasonally available produce is one way to help keep our bodies healthy and in sync with the naturally occurring biological rhythms of the seasons.

» Try to eat from every color category on the Rainbow Food Chart (figure 6) each day.

» Concentrate on getting plenty of fiber, by choosing fruits and vegetables which are higher in fiber, including foods from the prebiotic food list. (Figure 4)

» You need between 9-12 servings of whole, plant-based foods daily. A serving size is roughly ½ cup of raw or cooked vegetables, 1 cup of raw leafy greens, 1 cup of berries, 1 cup of cut fruit, or one medium sized piece of whole fruit. These healthy carbohydrates should make up about 30-35% of your daily calories.

» Have 3 servings of plant-based foods such as fresh fruits, vegetables, and dark leafy greens at each meal. Again, reference (figure 6) for ideas. Plant-based foods should cover about ¾ of your plate.

» Have a serving of protein at each meal. One serving of protein equates to ½ cup of beans/lentils (stage 3 only), 2-3 eggs; 3-6 ounces of fish, meat, or poultry; 2 tbsp. of nut butter, or ¼ cup of nuts/seeds.

» Protein should make up about ¼ of your plate. For most people, no more than 20-25% of your daily caloric intake should come from protein. Even athletes and body builders don't need more than 35%

» Healthy fats are unrestricted, and should make up relatively 40-50% of your daily caloric intake. Have at least one serving of healthy fat at each meal. One serving is approximately 1 tbsp. of oil, 2 tbsps. of nuts, 1 tbsp. of nut or seed butter, or 1/3 of an avocado.

» Be careful to store your oils in a cool, dark area, to prevent them from degrading. Only buy quantities that you can use in a reasonable amount of time. This way, your oils are always fresh.

» Don't cook with oil on high heats. This can damage the oil and cause it to become unhealthy. So, for example: stir frying over a medium/low heat is fine, but deep frying or frying on a high heat is not.

» Since over-cooking vegetables can cause them to lose some of their valuable nutrients and fiber content, try to eat raw vegetables when you can, and keep your cooked vegetables a little on the al dente side.

» Have 2-3 servings of fresh fruit, daily. A serving is generally 1 cup of berries, 1 cup of cut fruit, or one medium sized piece of whole fruit.

» Don't drink fruit juices, such as apple juice or orange juice. Fruit juices often contain added sugars, and even 100% juice blends are just concentrated forms of sugar. This is because it can take up to six pieces of fruit to make an 8-ounce glass of juice. That's six times more sugar than is found in a single piece of fruit. Moreover, since juice lacks the beneficial fiber contained in a whole piece of fruit, absorption of all that sugar will occur in minutes, effectively causing sugar and insulin spikes in your blood.

» Save dairy products for an occasional snack or treat.

» Have up to 1 ounce of dark chocolate (containing 72% or more cocoa) daily.

» Grains, sweet potatoes, yams, beans, and starchy vegetables are all interchangeable. A half cup is the serving size for one serving of grains, beans, or starchy vegetables. You can have up to two servings of these foods daily. (**Stage 3 only**)

» Eat a high-protein meal for breakfast. This will help keep your blood sugar level, and give you the energy to get through the morning without being hungry.

STAGE 2, THE ABLE BODY - FOODS LIST

Vegetables to choose often:

(Try to include 3 servings with every meal)

- » Dark leafy greens, such as spinach, kale, beet greens, collards, mustard greens, chard, dandelion greens, romaine, arugula, micro greens, etc.
- » Mushrooms
- » Peppers of all kinds
- » Tomatoes
- » Cucumbers
- » Onions
- » Leeks
- » Scallions
- » Garlic
- » Fennel
- » Celery
- » Zucchini and yellow squash
- » Spaghetti squash
- » Eggplant
- » Turnips and rutabagas
- » Carrots
- » Radishes
- » Pumpkin
- » Cruciferous vegetables, such as broccoli, cauliflower, cabbage, bok choy, and Brussels sprouts
- » Sprouts
- » Asparagus
- » Bamboo shoots

» Artichokes

» Green beans

» Kohlrabi

» Broccoli rabe

» Okra

» Water chestnuts

» Snow peas

» Jicama

» Raw beets

Vegetables to avoid:

» Potatoes

» Corn

» Acorn squash

» Cooked beets

» Peas

» Plantains

» Butternut squash

» Yams

» Sweet potatoes

» Parsnips

Fruits to choose often

(2-3 daily)

» Berries, such as blueberries, raspberries, black berries, and strawberries

» Apples

» Pears

- » Apricots
- » Nectarines
- » Peaches
- » Plumbs
- » Citrus, such as oranges, grapefruit, tangerines, lemons, and limes
- » Fresh figs
- » Kiwi
- » Cherries
- » Cranberries

Fruits to avoid:
- » Mango
- » Papaya
- » Pineapple
- » Banana
- » Red, black, and green grapes
- » Melon, such as watermelon, cantaloupe, and honeydew
- » Dried fruit, dates, and raisins
- » Fruit juice

Fats to choose often:
(Include healthy fats at all meals)
- » Avocado
- » Organic extra virgin coconut oil
- » Flaxseed oil
- » Extra virgin olive oil
- » Sesame oil

- » Whole flaxseed
- » Flax meal
- » Chia seeds
- » Hemp seeds
- » Pumpkin seeds
- » Sesame seeds
- » Sunflower seeds
- » Seed butters
- » Nuts, such as almonds, walnuts, pistachios, pecans, Brazil nuts, hazelnuts, peanuts, and cashews
- » Nut butters, like peanut, almond, and cashew
- » HBC mayo (See recipe section)
- » Mayo without added sugar, sweeteners, artificial sweeteners, or unhealthy oils
- » Grass-fed butter

Fats to choose less often:
- » Heavy cream
- » Half & Half
- » Sour cream
- » Cheese

Fats to avoid:
- » Trans fats (fats that are partially or fully hydrogenated)
- » Processed vegetable oils, like soy bean oil, sunflower oil, corn oil, canola oil, cottonseed oil, or safflower oil

Choose full fat dairy for an occasional snack or treat (serving size = 1/2 cup, or 1 oz. of cheese)

- » Plain Greek yogurt – a good source of protein and probiotics
- » Kefir – a good source of probiotics
- » Cottage cheese – a good source of protein
- » Cheese

Proteins

(1 serving at every meal)

- » 2-3 whole eggs
- » 3-6 ounces of poultry
- » 3-6 ounces of red meat, such as grass-fed beef, grass fed lamb, or pork; or wild game, like bison, elk, or venison
- » 3-6 ounces of wild fish, such as sardines, salmon, light tuna, cod, lake trout, halibut, or shellfish (at least 2x a week)
- » 2 tbsp. of nut butter
- » 1/4 cup of nuts or seeds

Fermented foods, choose often

(look for varieties which have been cured in salt, and which do not contain added sugar)

- » Fermented pickles
- » Sauerkraut
- » Kimchi
- » Fermented vegetables

Choose fresh or dried, herbs and spices as often as possible

- » Fresh ginger and turmeric

» Powdered ginger, turmeric, and cumin

» Fresh or dried basil, rosemary, oregano, dill, cilantro, thyme, and parsley

» Garlic powder, black pepper, cayenne pepper, paprika, coriander, cardamom, cinnamon, ancho chili, and other spices.

» 100% raw cacao powder

Condiments to choose often

» Vinegar

» Salsa without added sugar, sweeteners, or artificial sweeteners

» Hot sauce

» Marinara and tomato sauces without added sugar, sweeteners, or artificial sweeteners

» Pesto sauce

» Full fat dressings without added sugar, sweeteners, or artificial sweeteners

» Plain or spicy mustards without added sugar, sweeteners, or artificial sweeteners

» Gluten free soy sauce/tamari sauce

» Healthy Body Connection marinades and dressings (See recipe section)

» HBC Mayo (See recipe section)

» Guacamole

» Olive oil

Condiments to avoid

» Ketchup with added sugar, sweeteners, or artificial sweeteners

» BBQ sauce

- » Low-fat dressings
- » Dressings, marinades, dips, and sauces with sugar, sweeteners, or artificial sweeteners
- » MSG
- » Soy sauce

Avoid all added sugars, sweeteners, and artificial sweeteners, such as: (including Healthy Body Connection recipes with any added sweeteners)

- » Date sugar
- » Agave
- » Barley malt
- » Brown & white sugar
- » Cane juice
- » Corn syrup
- » Dextrose
- » Dextran
- » Florida crystals
- » Fructose
- » Juice concentrate
- » Glucose
- » Grape sugar
- » High fructose corn syrup
- » Honey
- » Hydrolyzed starch
- » Maltodextrin
- » Maltose
- » Maple syrup
- » Molasses

» Rice syrup

» Sucrose

» Turbinado sugar

» Palm coconut sugar

» Coconut sugar

Have daily if desired

» Dark chocolate (containing 72% or more cocoa,) 1 ounce daily.

STAGE THREE - THE DAILY CONNECTION STAGE

Congratulations, you have made it to stage 3, the Daily Connection! Although this is the last stage of the plan, the Daily Connection is the beginning of many wonderful things to come. This is the stage where you learn to listen to what your body is telling you. You'll pay careful attention for clues and insights on how your body is reacting to certain foods, so that you can customize the plan to fit your personal needs. This is also when you'll begin to incorporate other positive lifestyle changes into your daily life, so that you can fully maximize your results!

Let's begin this part of your journey by discussing the dietary aspects, first. In the Daily Connection stage, you may add whole grains, starchy vegetables, and other items, such as higher glycemic fruits, back into your diet. Grains, sweet potatoes, yams, beans, and starchy vegetables are all interchangeable. A ½ cup is the serving size for one serving of grains, starchy vegetables, or beans. You can have up to two servings of these foods daily.

When including grains back into your daily food plan, I would recommend starting with gluten-free grains like quinoa and gluten-free steel cut oats for the first week, at least. After that, if you choose, you can carefully begin to incorporate other whole grains back into your diet, always paying careful attention to how your body reacts to each new addition.

In addition to the dark chocolate, at this time you may also have up to 2 tsp/8g of added sugar, daily. I prefer that you limit your sugar products to raw honey, pure maple syrup, and organic coconut sugar. Be aware of how much added sugar you are eating each day, and avoid going over the 2 tsp/8g limit.

You may also enjoy an alcoholic beverage from time to time, if you wish. Although 1-2 drinks a day is alright, aim to make your alcohol intake more *occasional* than habitual. Remember that, for some of you, alcohol consumption may interfere with your weight loss/health goals, and you may need to abstain from drinking alcoholic beverages for a while.

FOR PRE-DIABETICS AND THOSE WITH TYPE 2 DIABETES

If you have a strong family history of chronic illness or type 2 diabetes; if you have been told by your doctor that you are pre-diabetic, insulin resistant; or if you already have type 2 diabetes: you may want to stay on a modified version of Stage 2, the Able Body stage.

As per the National Institute of Diabetes and Digestive and Kidney Diseases, "*People with a fasting glucose level of 100 to 125 mg/dL have impaired fasting glucose (IFG), or prediabetes. A level of 126 mg/dL or above, confirmed by repeating the test on another day, means a person has diabetes.*" Both the American Diabetes Association and the Mayo Clinic recommend that target blood glucose levels for individuals who have diabetes should generally range between 80mg/dl – 130mg/dl.

A close friend, who I'll call Ken, was recently diagnosed by his doctor as being pre-diabetic. In truth, his numbers were high enough, often enough, to be considered diabetic by the National Institute of Diabetes and Digestive and Kidney Diseases. We've found that the best way for him to control his blood sugar is by eating a well-balanced, low glycemic, high fiber diet. He avoids eating sugar, grains, and potatoes. He eats a varied whole foods diet, which includes protein, healthy fats, low glycemic fruits (like berries,) and lots of non-starchy vegetables. By following these guidelines, it only took Ken a few weeks to bring his fasting blood sugar (which was often above 180 mg/dl,) consistently down to below 90 mg/dl. The best part is, he has accomplished this miracle without taking any diabetes medications at all!

For those of you who fall into this category, enjoy your daily ounce of dark chocolate, limit your added sugar to 2 tsp/8g or less per day, and avoid eating grains, and potatoes. If you'd like even tighter control over your blood sugar, you can try limiting or omitting the intake of legumes and starchy vegetables as well.

An alternate approach for regulating your blood sugar would be to test how well your body tolerates specific foods, by checking your blood glucose levels one hour after eating. You can use this information to compare how certain foods affect your blood sugar, in contrast to meals without them.

I'd like to note that any significant changes toward a healthier diet will result in an improved outcome for most people. However, for people with blood sugar issues or a strong family history of chronic disease, a lower glycemic diet is going to be one of the most effective ways to take back the power over your own body, and promote your own good health.

FOR EVERYONE

As human beings, we all share a need for certain nutrients, and some things are just unhealthy for us all, but, because we are all individuals with different biological makeups, what is ideal for me may not be optimal for you. For example, while many people can thrive on a very low carbohydrate diet, there are just as many who would burn out and crash following the same regime; and there are those who can flourish with a lot more fat in their diets than others can even tolerate.

This plan sets you up with a solid foundation of information, and the basic guidelines of a healthy diet. Do your best, and remember that everything doesn't always have to be perfect or exact. The point is not to obsess over tracking ratios, but to find a healthy way of eating that is right for you. Maybe you need a few more carbs. Maybe you feel better with a bit more fat. Maybe you can't tolerate even a little dairy. Pay attention to how you're feeling, and what your body is telling you. Start out with the Daily Connection food plan, and tweak it over time to make it the best plan for you.

Now, it's also going to be very important to notice how specific foods affect your body as you begin to add them back into your diet. Add back one kind of food at a time, and see how you feel over the next 48 hours. Be on the lookout for any foods which cause increased cravings and hunger, stomach ache, bloating, gassiness, lethargy, headache, muscle or joint pain, soreness, runny nose, nausea, skin rashes, or diarrhea.

If you find that your body reacts adversely to any individual food, avoid that food for a while and see how you react to it again in a week or two. If at that point you find this food still causes you discomfort, consider eliminating it from your diet.

Remember, do the best you can. There is no need to obsess over the numbers. The most important part is to focus on eating a varied and nutrient-dense diet. If you only got in 6 plant-based foods today, or ate an extra piece of fruit, don't stress about it; tomorrow is another day, and another chance to do even better.

You are making a wondrous lifestyle change, a change that is going to make your life, and probably the lives of your friends and family, better and happier. Celebrate the fact that you are already on the path to better health and a longer life!

STAGE 3, THE DAILY CONNECTION - FOODS LIST

Vegetables to choose often:

(Try to include 3 of these with every meal)

» Dark leafy greens such as spinach, kale, beet greens, collards, mustard greens, chard, dandelion greens, romaine, arugula, micro greens etc.

- » Mushrooms
- » Peppers of all kinds
- » Tomatoes
- » Cucumbers
- » Onions
- » Leeks
- » Scallions
- » Garlic
- » Fennel
- » Celery
- » Zucchini and yellow squash
- » Spaghetti squash
- » Eggplant
- » Turnips and rutabagas
- » Carrots
- » Radishes
- » Pumpkin
- » Cruciferous vegetables such as broccoli, cauliflower, cabbage, bok choy, and Brussels sprouts
- » Sprouts
- » Asparagus
- » Bamboo shoots
- » Artichokes
- » Green beans
- » Kohlrabi
- » Broccoli rabe
- » Okra
- » Water chestnuts

» Snow peas

» Jicama

» Raw beets

Starchy vegetables & grains to choose less often
(Up to 2 x daily)

» Acorn squash

» Beets

» Peas

» Parsnips

» Plantains

» Butternut squash

» Yams

» Sweet potatoes

» Purple potatoes

» Beans

» Whole grains, such as quinoa, steel cut oats, farro & bulgur

Starchy vegetables & grains foods to avoid:

» White potatoes

» Corn

» Rice

Optional grains to avoid:

Increasingly, people are finding they have a gluten sensitivity these days. Gluten is known to cause inflammation, and some doctors feel that gluten may contribute to the loss of integrity of the intestinal protective lining, which can lead to serious illness. If you would like to go gluten free, see (figure 3) on page 52, for a list of foods that contain gluten.

Fruits to choose often

(2-3 daily)

» Berries, such as blueberries, raspberries, black berries, and strawberries

» Apples

» Pears

» Apricots

» Nectarines

» Peaches

» Plumbs

» Citrus fruits, such as oranges, grapefruits, tangerines, lemons, and limes

» Fresh figs

» Kiwi

» Cherries

» Cranberries

Fruits to choose less often:

(These fruits are higher on the glycemic index, and should only be eaten occasionally)

» Mango

» Papaya

» Pineapple

» Banana

» Melon, such as watermelon, cantaloupe, and honeydew

» Dried fruit, dates, and raisins (1-2 tbsp)

» Red or black grapes

Fats to choose often:

(Include healthy fats at all meals)

» Avocado

» Organic extra virgin coconut oil

» Flax seed oil

» Extra virgin olive oil

» Sesame oil

» Whole flaxseed

» Ground flaxseed

» Chia seeds

» Hemp seeds

» Pumpkin seeds

» Sesame seeds

» Sunflower seeds

» Seed butters

» Nuts, like almonds, walnuts, pistachios, pecans, Brazil nuts, hazelnuts, and cashews

» Peanuts

» Nut butters like peanut, almond, and cashew

» HBC mayo (See recipe section)

» Mayo without added sugar, sweeteners, artificial sweeteners, or unhealthy oils

» Grass-fed butter

Fats to choose less often:

» Heavy cream

» Half & Half

» Sour cream

» Cheese

Fats to avoid:

» Trans fats (fats that are partially or fully hydrogenated)

» Processed vegetable oils, like soy bean oil, sunflower oil, corn oil, canola oil, cottonseed oil, or safflower oil

Choose full fat dairy for an occasional snack or treat

(serving size= 1/2 cup or 1 oz. of cheese)

» Plain Greek yogurt – a good source of protein and probiotics

» Kefir – a good source of probiotics

» Cottage cheese – a good source of protein

» Cheese

Proteins -1 Serving at Every Meal

» 2-3 whole eggs

» 3-6 ounces of poultry

» 3-6 ounces of red meat, such as grass-fed beef, grass-fed lamb, or pork; or wild game, like bison, elk, or venison

» 3-6 ounces of wild fish, such as sardines, salmon, light tuna, cod, lake trout, halibut, or shellfish (at least 2x a week)

» 2 tbsp of nut butter

» 1/4 cup of nuts or seeds

» ½ cup of beans or lentils

Fermented foods, choose often (look for varieties which have been cured in salt, and which do not contain added sugar)

» Fermented pickles

» Sauerkraut

» Kimchi

» Fermented vegetables

Choose fresh or dried, herbs and spices as often as Possible

» Fresh ginger and turmeric

» Powdered ginger, turmeric, and cumin

» Fresh or dried basil, rosemary, oregano, dill, cilantro, thyme, and parsley

» Garlic powder, black pepper, cayenne pepper, paprika, coriander, cardamom, cinnamon, ancho chili, and other spices.

» 100% raw cacao powder

Condiments to choose often

» Vinegar

» Salsa without added sugar, sweeteners, or artificial sweeteners

» Hot sauce

» Marinara and tomato sauces without added sugar, sweeteners, or artificial sweeteners

» Pesto sauce

» Full fat dressings without added sugar, sweeteners, or artificial sweeteners

» Plain or spicy mustards without added sugar, sweeteners, or artificial sweeteners

» Gluten-free soy sauce

» Healthy Body Connection marinades and dressings (See recipe section)

» HBC mayo (See recipe section)

» Guacamole

Condiments to choose less often

» HBC ketchup (See recipe section)

Condiments to avoid

» Ketchup with added sugar, sweeteners, or artificial sweeteners

» BBQ sauce

» Low-fat dressings

» Dressings, marinades, dips, and sauces with sugar, sweeteners, or artificial sweeteners

» MSG

Have daily if desired

» Dark chocolate (containing 72% or more cocoa,) 1 ounce daily.

CHAPTER 7

VITAMINS, MINERALS, AND SUPPLEMENTS

A word of caution: whereas, almost anybody can benefit by taking a good multi vitamin, be very careful when choosing to take additional vitamins, minerals, antioxidants, or herbal supplements.

It might surprise you to know but there are a few irresponsible, celebrity doctors who use their books and their websites, to extol the multiple health benefits of every available form of supplementation known to mankind, from antioxidants and vitamins, to minerals and ancient herbal extracts. They make bold statements and promise you that these products will give you more energy, balance your hormones, improve your memory, speed up your metabolism, and help you lose weight, all while improving the quality of your sleep, your hair, and your skin! What's not surprising is that many of these same doctors have convenient online drug stores where you can easily purchase these miracle products with a simple mouse click and your credit card.

Now, I'm not saying that taking a supplement is a bad idea. Many people do benefit from various types of supplementation. What I am saying is that these hot shot doctors never take the time to tell you about the harmful side effects which have the potential to make you very sick.

Side effects which can cause everything from stomach upset, and diarrhea, to seizures.

Did you know that taking increased dosages of certain vitamins can cause deficiencies in others? Or that some supplements can interfere with the medications that you're taking? There are even a few supplements which cannot be safely combined with *other* supplements.

In addition, supplements can change the way your body works. They can thin your blood, lower your blood pressure, and effect on the hormone levels in your body. You need to know this kind of information before taking something new. What if you're already on a blood thinner, or medication to lower your blood pressure? What if you're on hormone replacement therapy? How could these supplements effect your health? If that weren't bad enough, many of them can worsen conditions, like kidney disease, liver disease, and diabetes. Imagine how tragic that could be for someone who unknowingly speeds up the progression of an already treacherous disease by taking something they thought would help them get healthier?

It's so important to do your homework. Be cautious of bold claims that don't give you all the information. Make sure you thoroughly research any new vitamin, mineral, antioxidant, or herbal remedy that you're thinking about trying. Investigate all the possible interactions and side effects. Remember to always ask your own doctor for their advice, before taking anything new - no matter how wonderful it sounds.

SOME SUPPLEMENTS TO ASK YOUR DOCTOR ABOUT

As I said earlier, many people do derive health benefits by taking supplements. For a bunch of different reasons such as: diet, physical condition, and medications, there are also lots of people who have vitamin and mineral deficiencies that they may not even be aware of. The health implications for these deficiencies can be serious. That's why in "The Healthy Start" (stage one), I recommend getting tested.

I'd like to break it down, and discuss some of the various vitamins, minerals, and supplements which may be of benefit. I'll include information on the possible side effects and interactions that I'm aware of, but again I urge you to check with your doctor and get their advice *before* taking anything new. Your doctor can verify if a specific supplement would be useful to you personally, and if it would be safe with your specific medical background taken into consideration. He or she can also recommend the dose which would best work for you.

ALPHA-LIPOIC ACID

Alpha-Lipoic Acid is a natural occurring antioxidant compound that is made in small amounts in the body. It is both water and fat soluble, which means it is used throughout the body. Alpha-lipoic acid has been shown to reduce blood sugar levels, improve insulin sensitivity, and to be useful in treating peripheral diabetic neuropathy (a condition which causes pain, burning, itching and numbness due to diabetic nerve damage). It has also been suggested that alpha-lipoic acid, may protect the brain from stroke and possibly dementia.

A 2011 study published in the American Journal of Medicine, concluded that giving obese subjects oral doses of alpha-lipoic acid was effective in achieving significant weight loss, and that it may potentially be useful as an adjunctive medication for obesity.

Side effects are generally rare and may include: insomnia, fatigue, nausea, vomiting, diarrhea, itchiness, and skin rash. It is unknown if alpha-lipoic acid is safe for women who are pregnant or nursing. Alpha-lipoic acid is not recommended for pediatric use.

Possible interactions:

» Medications for diabetes: Alpha-lipoic acid can lower blood sugar. Always consult your doctor before taking any supplements. Your doctor will need to monitor you carefully and adjust your medications to prevent hypoglycemia (dangerously low blood sugar levels).

» Chemotherapy medications

» Thyroid medications: Alpha-lipoic acid may lower levels of thyroid hormones. Again, check with your doctor before beginning to take any supplements.

» Vitamin B1 (thiamine): Alpha-lipoic acid can lower the level of vitamin B1 in the body. This can be dangerous for those who are already suffering from malnutrition, or in people who drink in excess.

ASHWAGANDHA (WITHANIA SOMNIFERA)

Ashwagandha is one of the most highly regarded herbs used in Ayurveda, an ancient form of holistic medicine which has been practiced in India for thousands of years. It's considered to be a powerful adaptogen (a natural substance considered to help the body adapt to stress and to exert a normalizing effect upon bodily processes,) and it's often used to help treat cancer, diabetes, stress, fatigue, and hypothyroidism. It is purported to help promote health, energy, strength, and memory, and has also been found useful in treating neurodegenerative diseases like Parkinson's and Alzheimer's disease.

Warnings: Pregnant and nursing women should not take Ashwagandha. The safety of this herb to infants is unknown. Ashwagandha may induce miscarriage in pregnant women.

Side effects: Large doses may cause stomach upset, vomiting and diarrhea. Ashwagandha can irritate the gastrointestinal tract – don't take Ashwagandha if you have a stomach ulcer.

Possible interactions:

» Sedatives: Ashwagandha may increase sedative effects, avoid taking Ashwagandha with sedatives.

» Medications for diabetes: Ashwagandha may lower blood sugar. Always consult your doctor before taking any supplements. Your doctor will need to monitor you carefully and adjust your medications to prevent hypoglycemia (dangerously low blood sugar levels).

» Blood pressure: Ashwagandha may lower blood pressure levels. This could cause blood pressure to drop to dangerously low for people with low blood pressure or for people who are on blood pressure medications. Again, check with your doctor before taking any supplements.

» Auto-immune diseases: Ashwagandha may cause the immune system to become more active. Don't use Ashwagandha if you have an autoimmune disease.

» Surgery: Ashwagandha slows the central nervous system and may interact with anesthesia and other medications normally associated with surgery. Stop taking Ashwagandha at least 2 weeks before a scheduled surgery.

» Thyroid medications: Ashwagandha may increase levels of thyroid hormones. If you are on any thyroid medications, use caution and check with your doctor before taking Ashwagandha.

VITAMIN B COMPLEX

Vitamin B complex is a vitamin supplement which contains 6 or more of the essential B vitamins. B vitamins are required for the maintenance and control of many biological functions such as: energy production, brain function, memory, concentration, and DNA synthesis. These vitamins also play a role in promoting mental health and cardiovascular health. They have been shown to protect against cancer, morning sickness, and the symptoms of premenstrual syndrome too.

I started taking vitamin B complex on the advice of my physician to help me with premenstrual syndrome which for me, included a premenstrual brain fog. The onset of my cycle always came with what I called, "a case of the premenstrual dumbs." I'd find myself having difficulty focusing, and making mistakes at work. It was embarrassing and frustrating. It felt like the harder I tried not to make mistakes, the worse it would get. I can attest that the vitamins helped. I still make mistakes sometimes, but I haven't had "a case of the premenstrual dumbs" in over six years.

Side effects: Side effects are uncommon when taking the proper dosage. Mild upset stomach or flushing may occur. Taking excessive amounts of Vitamin B complex can cause side effects. Signs of an overdose are: dizziness, frequent urination, a change in urine color (vitamin B2/Riboflavin frequently turns urine a bright yellow-orange color and is not a cause for alarm), black stools, constipation, diarrhea, abdominal pain, nausea, vomiting, redness of the skin, and itching.

Warnings: Though it is rare, some people can develop an allergic reaction to their vitamin B complex. If you develop symptoms of an allergic reaction such as: a rash, itching or swelling, dizziness, or trouble breathing, get medical help immediately.

You should not take B vitamin supplements if you are pregnant, nursing, suffer from diabetes, ulcers, gout, or if you are prone to allergic reactions. The use combination of vitamin B12, folate and vitamin B6 may increase the risk of blood vessel narrowing, do not take this combination after receiving a coronary stent. Before taking any new supplements or medications, always check with your doctor for the correct dosage and to make sure there will be no adverse interactions with any other medications or supplements which you may already be taking.

VITAMIN B12

Due to diet, medications, or medical conditions, many people are deficient in vitamin B12. Vitamin B12, also called cobalamin, is one of the 8 essential B vitamins. The human body need vitamin B12 to make red blood cells, nerves, and DNA. Vitamin B12 works with folic acid to help iron to work better in the body and to produce S-adenosylmethionine, (SAMe). SAMe is a chemical found in the body which is involved in both immune function and mood. Vitamin B12 supplementation may be useful in the prevention of breast cancer, and age related macular degeneration. It has traditionally been used as part of the treatment for: male infertility, chronic fatigue syndrome, heart disease, and hypothyroidism. Vitamin B12 is also believed to help improve: memory, concentration, and mood. Since B vitamins work symbiotically, you may want to take your B12 with other B vitamins. Vitamin B12 is found naturally in food sources such as: meat, poultry, fish, dairy and eggs.

People who are at risk for a vitamin B12 deficiency are:

» Vegans and vegetarians

» People with digestive disorders

» People who have been taking acid blocking medications for an extended period

» Heavy drinkers

» People who've had weight loss surgery

» People with diabetes

» The elderly

» People with HIV

» People with eating disorders

» People with pernicious anemia – a condition where your body cannot absorb vitamin B12

» The symptoms of a vitamin B12 deficiency are:

» Fatigue

» Weakness

» Lightheadedness

» Jaundice

» Heart palpitations

» Shortness of breath

» Pale skin

» Weight loss

- » Loss of appetite
- » Difficulty maintaining balance
- » Constipation, diarrhea, gas, and loss of appetite
- » Nervousness, and confusion
- » Memory loss, depression, and moodiness
- » Dementia
- » Soreness of the mouth or tongue
- » Numbness, and tingling sensations in the fingers and toes

Side effects: Vitamin B12 is considered safe and non-toxic.

Possible interactions: Vitamin B 12 can interact with certain medications and certain medications may adversely affect vitamin B12 levels. Individuals taking medication should discuss their vitamin B12 status with their healthcare providers. Some of the medications which may interact adversely with vitamin B12 are antibiotics like, Chloramphenicol and Tetracycline.

Other medications may interfere with vitamin B12 absorption, such as the following:

- » Anti-seizure medications like, Dilantin, Phenobarbital, and Mysoline
- » Chemotherapy medications, particularly Methotrexate
- » Proton pump inhibitors, like Omeprazole, and Lansoprazole
- » H2 receptor antagonists, medications like Tagamet, Pepcid, and Zantac
- » Diabetes medications like, Metformin

Warning: Do not take vitamin B12 if you have Leber's disease. It can seriously harm the optic nerve and could lead to blindness. Due to the possible harmful side effects, do not attempt to treat megaloblastic anemia with vitamin B12, without the close supervision of your physician. The use combination of vitamin B12, folate and vitamin B6 may increase the risk of blood vessel narrowing, do not take this combination after receiving a coronary stent. Before taking any new supplements or medications, always check with your doctor for the correct dosage and to make sure there will be no adverse interactions with any other medications or supplements which you may already be taking.

VITAMIN D & CALCIUM

More than one source tells us that vitamin D deficiencies are becoming a global concern. This is due to the fact that vitamin D is not abundantly available from natural food sources. While it is found in fatty fish and eggs, we get most of our vitamin D through a chemical reaction which occurs when our skin is exposed to the ultraviolet B rays of the sun.

Nowadays, due to lifestyles and occupations which keep us mainly indoors, and the necessary use of sunscreen to prevent skin cancer, our bodies are not exposed to as much sunlight as they were in the past.

Getting enough Vitamin D is important because, vitamin D deficiency has been linked to many illnesses including: cancer, osteoporosis, autoimmune disease, hypertension, infectious diseases, and depression. A vitamin D 25-Hydroxy, Serum level of 32ng/ml-100ng/ml is considered to fall within the normal range. However, many doctors feel that range is to wide and to avoid disease, optimal serum levels should fall between 50ng/ml and 80ng/ml.

The best vitamin D supplement to take is vitamin D3 because it's identical to the form of vitamin D produced by the body. I personally take 4000 IU of vitamin D3 daily, on the advice of my physician.

Most people don't experience any side effects to a vitamin D supplement. However, taking too much vitamin D can cause side effects which include:

» Excessive thirst

» Metallic taste in mouth

» Loss of appetite

» Weight loss

» Bone pain

» Tiredness

» Sore eyes

» Itchiness

» Vomiting

» Diarrhea

» Constipation

» Frequent urination

» Muscle pains

» Weakness

» Dry mouth

Ask your doctor for the correct dose for you.

People who have the following conditions should not take vitamin D unless under the direction of their physician:

» High blood calcium or phosphorous levels

» Kidney disease

» Atherosclerosis

» Sarcoidosis

» Histoplasmosis

» Hyperparathyroidism

» Lymphoma

» Tuberculosis

Possible interactions:

Vitamin D may interact adversely with several medications, including:

» Atorvastatin (Lipitor)

» Calcipotriene (Dovonex)

» Calcium channel blockers, such as: Nifedipine (Procardia), Verapamil (Calan, Covera, Isopin, verelan), Nicardipine (Cardene), Diltiazem (Cardizem, Dilacor, Tiazac) and Amlodipine (Norvasc)

» Digoxin (Lanoxin)

» Estrogen

» Isoniazid

» Water pills, such as: Thiazide, Chlorothiazide (Diuril), Hydrochlorothiazide, (HydroDiuril, Esidrix, Indapamide (Lozol), Metolazone (Zaroxolyn), and Chlorthialidone (Hygroton)

» Antacids

Calcium cannot be absorbed by the body without vitamin D. This in combination with dietary choices to avoid certain foods like dairy, may be the reason many Americans are also deficient in calcium. Calcium can be found in abundance from natural food sources such as: dairy products, almonds, salmon, broccoli, beans, greens, and sesame seeds. I see no need for calcium supplements, unless directed by your doctor. Getting enough vitamin D in combination with a balanced diet should give most people an adequate supply. Additionally, there has been some controversy over the efficacy and safety of taking calcium supplements.

MAGNESIUM

Magnesium is necessary to the function of more than 300 enzyme systems in the body, and is vital to protein synthesis, muscle and nerve function, blood glucose control, and blood pressure regulation.

Higher magnesium serum levels have been associated with better cardio vascular health, reduced risk of stroke, better blood glucose control in people with type 2 diabetes, and a reduced risk for osteoporosis. Magnesium supplements can be useful in treating depression, premenstrual syndrome, constipation, insomnia, and migraine headaches.

I began taking magnesium supplements to help with a recent development of premenstrual migraine headaches. My doctor advises me that these headaches are a perfectly normal occurrence at my age, due to the shifts in hormones prior to my cycle. Since starting on magnesium, I've noticed that my headaches are a lot less frequent, and when I do get a headache, they're a little less severe. As an added bonus, I find I sleep more deeply when I take my magnesium before bed.

Magnesium supplements are available in as many as nine different compounds. The most common are magnesium hydroxide, magnesium citrate, and magnesium sulfate. Magnesium hydroxide, and magnesium citrate are generally used as laxatives. Magnesium sulfate is available as Epson salts. Epson salts are used in a bath, allowing the magnesium to be absorbed by the skin. Epson salt baths are a relaxing way to help sooth sore muscles. Taking an Epson salt bath before bed will also help you to get a better night's sleep.

I choose to take my magnesium in the form of chelated magnesium glycinate. The body better absorbs this type of magnesium, it's less likely to have a laxative effect, and it's also known for having calming and relaxing properties.

Most people don't get enough magnesium from their diets. Adults need between 320 – 420mgs of magnesium daily, depending on sex and age. Some good dietary sources of magnesium include: Almonds, cashews, dark chocolate, peanuts, black beans, spinach, avocado, plain yogurt, bananas, broccoli, beets, and kidney beans. Other good sources include: milk, halibut, and chicken breast. Almonds come in the highest with 80mgs per one ounce serving, while chicken breast comes in at only 22mg per three ounces. Since only 30-40% of dietary magnesium is absorbed by the body, you would have to eat quite a bit of these kinds of foods to get an enough magnesium every day. Additionally, medical conditions and other factors can lead to lower levels of magnesium and magnesium deficiencies including:

» Gastro intestinal diseases and digestive disorders

» Diabetes

» Pancreatitis

» Hyperthyroidism (high thyroid hormone levels)

» Kidney disease

» Heavy menstrual periods

» Excessive sweating

» Drinking too much caffeine or alcohol

» Taking diuretics

» Taking steroids

» Prolonged stress

» Taking certain medications like; antibiotics, and chemotherapy drugs

» Prolonged use of proton pump inhibitors such as Omeprazole, Lansoprazole, and Esomeprazole (Prilosec, Prevacid & Nexium)

The symptoms of a magnesium deficiency include:

» Agitation and anxiety

» Restless leg syndrome

» Insomnia

» Nausea and vomiting

» Abnormal heart rhythms

» Low blood pressure

» Confusion

» Muscle spasm and weakness

» Seizures

» Head aches

Side effects: Common side effects for magnesium include, stomach upset, cramps, and diarrhea.

Warnings: People with heart or kidney disease should not take magnesium except as directed by their physician. Magnesium competes with calcium for absorption and can cause a calcium deficiency in people whose calcium levels are already low. Always check with your doctor for correct dosing and to see if taking magnesium makes sense for you. Overdosing on oral magnesium supplements can be very dangerous and can cause many serious health problems such as:

» Nausea

» Vomiting

» Very low blood pressure

» Confusion

» Muscle weakness

» Fatigue

» Slowed heart rate

» Respiratory paralysis

» Mineral deficiencies

» Cardiac arrhythmias

» Cardia arrest

» Coma

» Death

Possible interactions: Magnesium supplements may interact badly with other medications, such as:

» Aminoglycosides (a type of antibiotic), taking this medication while taking magnesium can cause neuromuscular weakness and paralysis

» Antibiotics – Nitrofurantoin and Quinolone antibiotics, magnesium should be taken 1 hour before or 2 hours after these types of antibiotics to avoid reducing the absorption of the medication. Quinolone antibiotics include: Ciprofloxacin, Moxifloxacin, Tetracycline, Doxycycline, and Minocycline.

» Blood pressure medications and calcium channel blockers in pregnant women: magnesium increase the risks of negative side effects from these medications in pregnant women.

» Diabetes medications: magnesium may increase the absorption of these medications. If you take these medications, your doctor may need to adjust your dose.

» Fluoroquinones: taking this medication while taking magnesium may decrease absorption and effectiveness. Fluoroquinones should be taken at least 4 hours before taking any products which contain magnesium.

» Hormone replacement therapy

» Labetol: taking this medication while taking magnesium can abnormally slow your heart beat and reduce cardiac output.

» Levomethadyl: taking this medication while taking magnesium may cause a heart condition.

» Levothyroxine: magnesium may reduce the effectiveness of this medication.

» Tiludronate and alendronate: magnesium should be taken 1 hour before or 2 hours after these types of osteoporosis medications to avoid reducing absorption of the medication.

PROBIOTICS

The internationally endorsed definition of probiotics is: live microorganisms that, when administered in adequate amounts, confer a health benefit on the host. Traditionally probiotics are used to treat or prevent an imbalance of the microflora which inhabit the intestines. New approaches have shown the potential for probiotics to be used as part of the treatment for a range of chronic diseases.

In a 2016 study, which was published in the journal BioMed Research International, Researchers in Italy studied 150 men to discern the efficacy of using probiotics in the treatment of Irritable Bowel Syndrome with constipation (IBS-C). In this study, a randomized, double blind, placebo controlled clinical trial, conducted over 2 years, scientists found that probiotics were effective in improving symptoms of IBS-C such as pain, flatulence, and bloating. Additionally, the decrease in constipation was twofold greater for participants who had been given probiotics in comparison to those who had been in the placebo group, and patients in the probiotic group reported an increased quality of life.

An imbalance in the intestinal microbiome leads to chronic intestinal inflammation which is characterized by a loss of integrity of the intestinal protective lining (the epithelial barrier), and an increase of inflammatory cytokines. Despite their differences, Crohn's disease, ulcerative colitis, and irritable bowel disease, are each characterized by the loss of epithelial barrier and increased production of inflammatory cytokines.

As a species, Lactobacillus are active against harmful bacteria, yeast, fungi, certain parasites, and viruses. However, in a 2016 Brazilian study, also published in the journal BioMed Research International, scientists were interested in the anti-inflammatory potential of a strain of Lactobacillus called Lactobacillus plantarum. In previous studies, Lactobacillus plantarum had been shown to decrease Helicobacter pylori activity, and to improve the symptoms of IBS. (Helicobacter pylori are a bacterium which are often associated with stomach infections and ulcers.) This time, researchers found that Lactobacillus plantarum, prevented pathogens from sticking to the epithelial barrier and significantly decreased the secretion of inflammatory cytokines. They concluded that Lactobacillus plantarum, had a strong anti-inflammatory effect on the protective intestinal barrier, and was a strong candidate to assist in therapy for inflammatory diseases.

In 2014, a three month, randomized, double blind, placebo controlled study, was published in the European Journal of Endocrinology. Researchers from the Diabetes and Metabolism, Rigshospitalet,

University of Copenhagen, studied the effects of Lactobacillus helveticus, on the glycemic control and cardiovascular risk factors of 41 men with type 2 diabetes. They divided the group of men randomly by a computerized system. One group received a yogurt fermented with 300ml of Lactobacillus helveticus, which they called Cardio4 yogurt. The other group received an identically formulated placebo yogurt which was fermented with an acidifier known as glucono-lactone, instead of the probiotic. The results were astounding. After 12 weeks of daily intake of the yogurt fermented with Lactobacillus helveticus, participants had a reduced average heart rate of 2 beats per minute, over 24 hours and in daytime. This is significant because, elevated heart rate is considered an important risk factor for cardio vascular disease. Additionally, Cardio4 yogurt reduced fasting plasma glucose levels, and scientists saw a trend towards improvement in insulin resistance in the probiotic group. Another bacteria called Bifidobacterium, is also known to reduce inflammation and improve glucose tolerance.

As research develops probiotic use is becoming more main stream. A study by the CDC, which was published in the American Journal of Infection Control, found that more and more patients are receiving probiotics as part of their inpatient hospital care. In fact, almost 3 times as many hospital patients were prescribed probiotics in 2012 as compared to patients in 2007.

Since the diversity and symbiosis of our microbiome is so intrinsically related to how are bodies are functioning, effecting everything from our immune systems, to our weight, mood, and sleep, maintaining it is an important aspect of our well-being. We can protect our microbiome by reducing stress, exercising, eating a healthy diet, and by taking a high-quality probiotic. Look for a probiotic which contains large amounts of many different species.

Side effects: Probiotics are considered be safe for healthy people. Most people do not experience any side effects. Rarely people may experience short term mild gas or bloating. If you are immune-compromised or have a serious illness, avoid taking probiotics unless your doctor has okayed their use. Probiotics should be used cautiously by pregnant women, infants, and young children. Never give probiotics to a premature infant.

RHODIOLA ROSEA

Rhodiola rosea is an adaptogen herb which grows at high altitudes in Siberia, the republic of Georgia, and Scandinavia. Because it grows in such a brutal climate, Rhodiola rosea is an amazing source of antioxidants. This astounding little yellow flower's roots, are attributed to conferring many health benefits. The list is amazingly long, and you might think a little too good to be true but, unlike many other such herbs, Rhodiola rosea has been studied extensively in the U.S. and abroad. Its many positive attributes have been well documented and are backed by scientific evidence. Rhodiola rosea has been proven to successfully: improve mood, increase stamina and athletic performance, improve weight loss and metabolism, improve brain function and memory, strengthen the immune system, safely relieve menopausal symptoms, and improve the bodies reaction to physical and mental stressors. The Soviet Union was aware of these benefits for years before we'd ever even heard of Rhodiola in America. They used it during the cold war to give their astronauts, athletes, soldiers, and scientists, a leading edge.

If you would like to try Rhodiola rosea, make sure you purchase from a reputable source. Many manufactures sell inferior products, which will not give you the desired effect. Look for a pure root extract which contains a minimum of 3% rosavins and 0.8% - 1.0% salidrosides. The product must only contain Rhodiola rosea and not a mix of Rhodiola species. Rhodiola rosea should be taken a half hour before eating for the best absorption, and should not be taken in the late afternoon as it may interfere with your sleep if taken to late in the day. It is usually best to take between 100 and 200 milligrams per day. Never take more than 400 milligrams a day without medical supervision.

Side effects:

» Rhodiola rosea in many ways acts as a stimulant. If you feel jittery or agitated after taking it you should cut back on the dosage you are taking, and build up to a higher dose gradually if you feel you need more. You can even open a capsule and only take ¼ or ½ of the regular dose.

» Some people experience intense dreams when they begin taking Rhodiola rosea, they should subside in about 2 weeks.

» Some people may experience nausea.

Warnings: Get your doctors approval before starting any new herbal products or supplements. Get your doctors approval before starting Rhodiola rosea if you suffer from manic episodes or bipolar disorder. People with these disorders would need close medical supervision while taking Rhodiola because of its stimulant like qualities. Don't take Rhodiola rosea if you are pregnant or breast feeding, since it is not known if it is safe for pregnant or breast-feeding women.

Interactions: Rhodiola rosea has not been shown to interact adversely with any prescription medications or other herbal products. Be aware that Rhodiola rosea may increase the stimulant action of other stimulants, or stimulant medications.

TULSI/HOLY BASIL

Tulsi (Ocimum sanctum) or Holy Basil is an herb from the basil family, and has been used in Ayurvedic Medicine for thousands of years. Like Ashwagandha, it's considered an adaptogen which helps the body adapt to stress and increases the body's resistance to disease. Tulsi has been used to treat colds, coughs, the flu, respiratory illness, fevers, headaches, stomach disorders, and heart disease. Its oils contain strong antioxidant and anti-inflammatory properties. Tulsi may be effective in helping people with type 2 diabetes in controlling their blood sugar.

Tulsi can be grown from seeds. Its leaves can be used similarly to other fresh herbs for use in recipes when cooking, or it can be seeped into a tea. The leaves can even be crushed into a paste which is used to treat skin infections, and as a fungicide. In India, many families grow Tulsi in their homes. In Hindu mythology, the plant is the incarnation of the goddess Tulsi and confers divine protection. Tulsi is also available as packaged tea, in powdered form, and as capsules and tablets.

Since fresh Tulsi is not readily available in my area, I buy Tulsi tea. The tea comes in a variety of flavors, it's caffeine free, and it can be served hot or iced. I've personally found Tulsi tea to be very soothing. I enjoy a cup anytime I want to relax and unwind.

Warning: Studies have found that large doses of Tulsi/Holy Basil may affect fertility negatively.

Interactions: There aren't many known interactions between this supplement and other medications. However, there are some concerns that Holy Basil may interact with Pentobarbital causing excessive drossiness, and with anti-coagulant medications, such as Aspirin and Warfarin, causing increased chances of bruising and bleeding.

If you are taking any medications, check with your doctor before taking Tulsi/Holy Basil.

CHAPTER 8

LIFESTYLE STRATEGIES

Earlier I covered some of the important aspects of how sleep, exercise, and stress can impact your hormones and your overall health. I discussed how too much stress and cortisol contribute to belly fat, hormonal imbalances, sleep disorders, and metabolic syndrome, and about how sleep deprivation can lead to weight gain, inflammation, and chronic illness. I also illustrated the importance of an active lifestyle and exercising to keep our mobility as we age, and to help protect us from diseases like cancer and coronary heart disease. I also included information on all the positive attributes of engaging in physical activities such as, improved mood, sleep, and insulin sensitivity.

Now, I'd like to touch on the topic of telomeres including, what they are, and how they relate to your health, longevity, and lifestyle.

Telomeres are the protective caps on the ends of our chromosomes, they have often been compared with the plastic tips on shoelaces, because they keep chromosome ends from fraying and sticking to each other.

Telomeres shorten a little bit each time a cell divides, and get shorter as we age. The length of our telomeres can affect both our health and our longevity. People with shorter telomeres age more rapidly and are more prone to diseases like: cancer, coronary heart disease, heart failure, diabetes, and osteoporosis. Having shorter telomeres has also been associated with having a shorter lifespan. There are many factors outside of normal aging which can prematurely shorten our telomeres. These include smoking, obesity, pollution, exposure to toxins, stress, and sleep deprivation.

Elizabeth H. Blackburn is a Nobel Laureate and Morris Hertzstein Professor of Biology and Physiology, in the Department of Biochemistry and Biophysics at the University of California San Francisco. She is a leader in the area of telomere research, and it was she, who discovered the molecular nature of telomeres.

In a 2015 study, which was published in the journal Molecular Psychiatry. Elizabeth H. Blackburn and a group of other esteemed researchers studied 239 healthy, non-smoking, post-menopausal women for one year. The study was developed to examine the effects that stress and stressful major life events would have on the length of the women's telomeres, and to see if lifestyle patterns played any role in the outcome. Major stressors in this study included: the death of a close friend or family member, extreme stress in the work place, loss of employment, financial burdens, being a caregiver, and troubled relationships. All things that most of us have experienced at one time or another. What they found was that major stressors over the year, significantly predicted accelerated telomere shortening over the same time period. In other words, too much stress might not give you gray hairs, but it can prematurely speed up the aging process.

Notably, they also found that women who maintained healthy lifestyles (a combination of eating a nutritious diet, getting enough sleep, and exercising,) had no telomere shortening when exposed to the same types of adverse life events. This proves once again, that our lifestyles can either be the predictors of illness, or of wellbeing.

The exciting news is that we can protect ourselves from early aging. We have the power to impact our hormones, our micro biome, and our genes.

HOW TO GET MOVING

Exercise. Many people groan inwardly just seeing or hearing the word because they think that for it to be effective, exercise has to be torture.

Additionally, to someone who's never been active before, the idea of exercise can be very intimidating. There can be uncertainty about how to begin, ability to participate, and how to be effective. I know a lot of people also equate exercising to joining a gym, and that's okay if going to a gym is something that you enjoy, but you don't have to join a gym to be healthy. The most important thing is that being active should be fun. It doesn't have to be torture, and it shouldn't be. How could anyone stick to doing an activity they hated?

You don't have to start big either. You can start by making a few small changes, and work your way up to being more active at your body's own pace. Here are some examples of things that you can do to get started:

» Park a little further from work, school, or the store

» Choose to take the stairs when you can

» Get up from your desk to walk around every hour or so

» Go for a walk on your lunch break

» Bike or walk to places whenever you can

» When you're at home find reasons to go up and down the stairs, or to walk from room to room

» Go for long walks after dinner with your favorite person

When I first began my own personal journey to better health, I bought a bicycle and a helmet, so that I could go for bike rides, and I bought an instructional DVD so I could learn to belly dance. I got moving in my own way, on my own terms, and I had fun doing it. You can too!

While we're on the topic, DVD's are a great resource. There's an abundance of different DVD's available, with professional trainers who'll guide you through an activity such as: dance, yoga, martial arts, weight training, or cardio. It's a no pressure way to becoming more active because you can work out in the privacy of your own home, at your own pace. You don't have to drive anywhere, and you can fit the activity into your own schedule, instead of rushing to keep an appointment. For many people, this is a great solution. I'm a certified personal trainer, capable of creating my own workouts, but I use DVD's all the time. I enjoy the convenience, the variety of activities available, and the personalities of the trainers. For me it can be more fun, and more motivating than working out on my own.

You need to be active for at least 30 minutes a day, 5-6 days a week, but fitting more movement into your life doesn't need to be hard core or extreme.

Here are a few more ideas to help you find an activity that's right for you. How about bike riding in the park, or dancing to your favorite tunes in your living room? What about taking a dance class, or a karate class, or joining a softball team? Maybe you like bowling, or have always wanted to learn to play tennis? Skiing, roller skating, canoeing, swimming, the possibilities are endless. Try something new, or perhaps rediscover an activity that you used to love. Getting your exercise can be a totally positive experience. Now is the time for you to find fun activities, and to enjoy your life!

GETTING ENOUGH SLEEP, THE MORE YOU KNOW...

It's fascinating to think about how all the key components of health: diet, sleep, exercise, and stress management, are all so interdependent on each other. For example, getting enough sleep at night helps us to better cope with stress during the day. Improved stress management helps us focus better and sleep better. Regular exercise during the day improves the quality of our sleep. Lack of sleep seems to cause increased hunger, especially for high calorie foods, and interestingly, what we eat may also affect how well we sleep!

In a 2016 study, published in the Journal of Clinical Sleep Medicine, researchers studied 26 healthy adults to see if diet could impact sleep.

They compared the sleep patterns of participants on a controlled high fiber diet, to the sleep patterns of the same participants when food choice was unrestricted. The results? When the participants ate a high fiber diet they slept better and more deeply, with less sleep disturbances. Conversely, when the participants consumed a low fiber - high sugar diet, they experienced a lest restful sleep, with more sleep disturbances.

Amazingly, the food we choose to eat can even affect the quality of our sleep! Many other things can too. Things like stress, our busy schedules, caffeine intake, and even our technology, can all interfere with our getting a good night's rest. More than one third of Americans don't get enough sleep, and when you think about how it all connects, getting enough sleep is one of the cornerstones of good health. Everyone is different, some people need a little less sleep than others, but on average most people require between 7 and 10 hours of sleep a night.

Here are some ideas to help you develop better sleep patterns:

1. Turn your bedroom into a peaceful oasis meant for sleep.

Keep your room dark, and cool. Remove all electronics from your room. Devices like televisions, phones, computers, and printers can all be too stimulating to allow you to relax, and the lights from these devices interfere with your sleep hormones. Make sure your bed and pillows are comfortable and that the room is well ventilated.

2. Set a regular sleep schedule.

Try to go to bed and wake up at the same time every day, even on weekends. Getting up at the same time every morning is the key, so try not to sleep in.

3. Try not to take naps.

Daytime naps can interfere with your nighttime sleep. If you do nap, try to make it before 3pm and nap for less than one hour.

4. Create a bedtime routine.

Those of us who are parents know how important a set bedtime with a quite bedtime routine is for getting small children to bed at night. The same rules apply to adults, maybe even more so. After our hectic, stressful, and hurried days, we need some down time to unwind and relax before bed if we want any chance at getting a peaceful night's sleep. Take an hour or two before bedtime each night to engage in some quite relaxing activities such as: reading, listening to some quite music, taking a warm bath, meditating, stretching, or practicing some relaxation yoga. Dim the lights to set a more sleep inducing atmosphere.

5. Try not to deal with anything too stressful or upsetting right before bed.

Strong negative emotions will keep you awake at night. You need to feel calm and relaxed to sleep.

6. Take notes or make a list for tomorrow.

In the evening, before you're too tired, write down everything that you want to remember for the next day. Keep this list near your bed, somewhere that you'll see it in the morning. By keeping it close by, you can add to it if you suddenly think of something else. When you're done you'll be better able to sleep because you won't be up all night, worrying about the things you must take care of tomorrow.

7. Don't keep looking at the time.

Once you're in bed don't play the how many hours' game. You know the one, if I fall asleep right now I'll get 6 hours, 4 hours, 3 hours... This just stresses you out, which can ruin your chances of getting any rest.

8. Limit your caffeine.

If you're having difficulty sleeping it could be that you're over caffein-ated. Limit your caffeine intake and don't have any caffeine late in the afternoon.

9. Don't drink alcohol to help you sleep.

Although alcohol may initially make you feel drowsy, it will interfere with and disrupt your sleep.

10. Exercise regularly, but not too close to bed time.

People who exercise sleep better, but exercising too late in the day can be too rousing. Remember you want to be relaxed, not invigorated before bed.

11. Don't eat a big meal too close to bedtime.

A big meal before bed will just make you uncomfortable and could interfere with your sleep. If you feel hungry before bed, have a small snack to satisfy your hunger.

12. Don't drink too much liquid an hour before bed.

Don't go to bed thirsty, but try not to drink too much right before bed. You don't want your sleep to be interrupted by added trips to the bathroom in the middle of the night.

13. Do keep some water near the bedside.

It's nice to have some fresh water handy for sipping if you should wake up with a dry throat or mouth, in the middle of the night.

14. Don't struggle.

Staying in bed when you can't sleep will only frustrate you and further prevent you from getting to sleep. If after 20 minutes or so you find that you can't fall asleep, get out of bed and go do something quite in another room. Although you may be tempted, *do not* use the time to catch up on work or your bills. You could become too awake and possibly too stressed, to get back in bed. Instead choose relaxing activities like reading, or listening to soft music.

15. Make the most out of the daylight.

Our bodies sleep patterns, are regulated by daylight. When you wake up in the morning open all the drapes and let the sun in. Get outside if you're able, and if it's dark when you arise, turn on all the lights.

SLEEP APNEA

If you snore loudly, awaken feeling unrested after a good night's sleep, awaken with a bad head ache, or a dry throat, you may have sleep apnea. Sleep apnea is a condition where breathing stops briefly during the night, sometimes several times during a night. Talk to your doctor if you think you have sleep apnea. Sleep apnea is a potentially dangerous condition which can lead to high blood pressure, type 2 diabetes, and non-alcoholic liver fatty liver disease. It also can increase the risks for stroke and sudden death.

RESTLESS LEG SYNDROME (RLS)

RLS is a neurological disorder which causes your legs to jerk or move at night. People who have RLS have an overwhelming urge to move or kick their legs, due to uncomfortable or painful sensations in their legs. The symptoms typically get worse at night when they are trying to relax or sleep.

PERIODIC LIMB DISORDER

Periodic limb disorder is a neurological disorder which causes a person's legs jump and twitch involuntarily every 20 to 40 seconds while they sleep.

There's an array of other medical conditions which can also interfere with your sleep such as: seasonal allergies, CODP, and depression. If you think you have a medical condition which is affecting your ability to sleep talk to your doctor.

TAKING A LOAD OFF

Most of us are living our lives under some sort of daily pressure. Whether it be problems at work, financial burdens, health issues, or just the stresses of everyday living; we all have things which happen in our lives that can make us feel worried, or cause us to feel stressed. This burden is not only a mental burden, but a physical one, which affects our bodies. Think about it, when we are stressed we get neck aches, stomach aches, and headaches. During a stressful encounter, our hearts can race and pound. Continual stress can also raise cortisol levels (which as mentioned previously causes inflammation,) the storage of belly fat, and can lead to a host of other health problems. Spending each day in a constant state of stress is like walking around with a crushing weight on your head and your shoulders all the time. How could anyone sleep, eat, enjoy relationships, or love their lives under such constant weight and pressure?

The answer lies in learning to take a load off. Not off your feet, but off your mind. Learning ways to better cope with unavoidable stress, to release or relieve stress, and to rid yourself of unnecessary stress, are how you take the load off.

SLEEP

I've already covered the importance of good sleep, and daily exercise so I'll just lightly touch on these two topics regarding how they can reduce your stress.

You've probably heard the expressions "everything will look better in the morning" and "let me sleep on it." That's because a good night's sleep really does put everything into perspective. Problems somehow loom larger than life, and things are harder to deal with when we are sleep deprived. Getting a good night's sleep is not only physically restorative, it's mentally restorative too. When we get enough sleep we are better able to make decisions, learn new stuff, remember things, and handle problems.

EXERCISE

Exercising creates endorphins, and endorphins make you happy. Endorphins are small chemical communicators produced by the body to alleviate pain. They also create feelings of euphoria and relaxation. That's why people feel happier after a good workout. Exercise also improves your blood flow, and helps bring more oxygen to your brain. Working out is a great way to blow off steam, relieve pent up stress, improve your focus, your mood, and help you to sleep better at night.

YOGA

Yoga, a form of exercise which has been around for about 5000 years, can be another great way to re-center yourself and relieve stress. The practice of yoga combines controlled breathing, strength, balance, and flexibility, with focus & serenity. The combination of physical activity and tranquility, really delivers when it comes to creating positive results. Practicing yoga can: lower your blood pressure, lessen anxiety, reduce depression, and diminish pain. Bonus benefits include: better balance and functionality in daily activities, increased muscle tone, improved range of motion, enhanced athletic performance, and a sense of well-being.

MEDITATION

You don't have to climb to the peak of the Himalayans, or become a Buddhist monk, to enjoy the inner peace that comes from practicing meditation.

Here's why you should try it. Meditation is one of the most powerful ways to elicit something known as "the relaxation response." The relaxation response is a physiological state of calmness, produced using relaxation techniques. There have been many benefits associated with creating this state of calmness. Regular meditation has been connected with: improved sleep, lower stress levels, better coping skills during stressful situations, a general feeling of wellbeing, improved brain function and focus, and a stronger immune system.

Additionally, meditation can have a positive effect on many health conditions which are often adversely affected by stress, such as: anxiety disorders, depression, high blood pressure, pain, asthma, acid reflux disease, and heart disease.

Keeping all of that in mind, here are seven easy steps to help you learn to meditate. Even if you don't do it regularly, these steps will help you to relax if you've had a very stressful day.

1. Set a low volume timer for 10 – 20 minutes.
2. Pick a word or phrase to repeat. This will be your mantra. It can be anything that makes you feel good, like "ocean breeze," "today is a good day," "happy," etc.
3. Sit in a quiet spot, in a comfortable position, with your eyes closed.
4. Relax all your muscles.
5. Breathe slowly and naturally. As you exhale, repeat your mantra silently to yourself. If other thoughts drift into your mind, it's okay. Just gently return to your mantra.
6. After the 10 – 20 minutes have passed, sit quietly for another minute or two and allow your thoughts to return.

7. Open your eyes and sit for another minute before rising, and resuming your regular activities.

There's also a variety of other meditation techniques that you can try. Single point or concentrative meditation, involves spending 10-20 minutes or more, focused on one object, sound, or image. You can focus on things like: a favorite photograph, a piece of art, soothing music, logs burning in a fire place, or a flower in the garden. It's normal for your mind to occasionally wander. If it does, just gently bring your focus back to your chosen object.

Another meditation technique which can be very affective, is guided meditation. In guided meditation, another person leads you through the meditation from beginning to end. Often such guided meditations are available as recordings, that you can listen to at home. If you think you'd enjoy trying some guided meditation, the UCLA Mindful Awareness Research center, and the Chopra Center, both offer some free voice guided meditations on their websites, http://marc.ucla.edu/ & http://www.chopra.com/articles/guided-meditations. You can also find many other sources for guided meditations like these, on the internet.

RELAXATION YOGA

Relaxation yoga is a series of gentle stretches meant to ease sore muscles and help calm your mind. Many people practice relaxation yoga before going to bed as part of their regular bedtime routine. You can listen to soft music while you move through the poses and you can even do some of the stretches right in your bed. Relaxation yoga is different than other forms of yoga. It isn't strenuous, and nearly anyone can participate. For a free demonstration please visit, http://healthybodyconnection.com/relaxation-yoga/

GET IN TOUCH WITH YOUR SURROUNDINGS

Whether it's a bare foot walk along the shore, or threw a grassy field, a walk through the woods on a fall day or just sitting enjoying the day for a few minutes in your own back yard, getting out into nature can be an excellent way to relieve your stress.

It might seem a little hokey, but it works. The trick is to use your time in nature to connect with your surroundings. Concentrate on the sights, sounds, smells, and sensations. Do you feel the sun on your face, or the breeze as it stirs around your skin? Can you feel the warm sand or soft grass beneath your feet? Do you hear birds calling in the trees, or the leaves crunching under your boots? Can you hear children laughing at play? Can you smell the sweetness of flowers in the wind? To notice the sights, sounds, and smells around you, you have to slow down enough to focus on them. This kind of open awareness, is actually another form of meditation, in which you are fully present and aware of all that is happening around you.

When I lived closer to the shore, I would often visit the beach. It was a small local beach which never had massive crowds of people on it. I would find myself a quiet spot to just sit and enjoy my surroundings. I'd watch the waves drift to the shore, and the seagulls as they flew, circled, and landed. I was aware of the other people on the beach like the children playing nearby, and the couples who were strolling on the shoreline. I could smell the salty ocean air. I could hear the cry of the gulls, the sound of the surf, and the laughter of the children. I can still remember clearly how the sun and breeze felt on my skin, and the feeling of the sand between my toes. I would instinctually go there whenever I needed some serenity and clarity. I would just sit there taking it all in. When I was ready to leave, I left feeling happy, serene, and rejuvenated.

I don't live near the ocean anymore, but I still practice this form of open awareness. Sometimes I go for a long walk. Sometimes I just sit in my yard enjoying the sun and the air. There is a true magic in noticing and appreciating the beauty of the world around you. It grounds you, and somehow at the same time it lifts you up.

DO THAT THING YOU LOVE DOING

Is there something that you love doing, that just feels natural and makes you happy?

What I'm talking about is that thing that you were born to do, that thing which fills you up inside. I like to call it your inner music, because it's like a beautiful song in your soul that needs to be expressed.

Almost anything can be the source of that inner music, from mountain climbing, to playing an instrument, from teaching, to quenching a thirst to learn. For some it could be the desire to create, to draw, cook, garden, or sculpt. For others, the music might be sharing their message, their truth, or their vision with others. The possibilities are unlimited, and it's something different for each of us. Whatever it is for you, it's important that you to make time in your life for it. Climb that mountain, write that book, reconnect with your creativity, open that dream business, or share your vision with the world.

Many of us put our own happiness on hold for someday, because we are just too busy or too bogged down by obligations today. The problem is that somehow, someday never arrives. By stifling your passions, you are editing yourself and denying the part of you that most makes you, you. You can't be truly happy, when you aren't being true to yourself. Don't stifle that special music within you. Follow your passions and live your best life today, tomorrow isn't guaranteed.

"Don't die with your music still in you"

- Dr. Wayne W. Dyer.

DON'T WORRY NEEDLESSLY

Happiness is the opposite of stress, and if you're worried you're not happy.

I always used to joke that I was born with the worry gene. I used to say that I inherited it from my grandmother. I adored my grandmother, she was kind, gentle, and loving, but she was a terrible worrier. I remember how when I was eight years old, she'd never let me go in more than a half inch of water when we'd visit the beach together. She'd keep a strong grip on my wrist, sure that I'd be swept out to sea by an undercurrent at any moment. I also remember how she'd nervously watch me, afraid that I'd fall and break both my legs, whenever she caught me walking along the foot-high brick borders which edged the trees and flower beds just outside of her apartment building. Her heart was in the right place I know, but she suffered needlessly from all of that worrying.

I might have actually inherited that gene, if there is such a thing. As I grew into an adult I found myself becoming increasingly fearful myself. I began to sweat the big stuff and the little stuff too. All that fear, and gut churning worrying was ruining my life. I spent years drowning in all that self-created misery. In time, I was fortunate enough to recognize what all that stress was doing to my life, my happiness, and my health. Intuitively, I began to make changes. Realizing that I had denied my true self for too long, I ended a stressful, and unfulfilling career path. I chose to take back my power, and to pursue my dreams. I started to learn that I didn't have to sweat so much of the small stuff.

Dr. Wayne Dyer was an internationally renowned author and motivational speaker. Often called the father of motivation, his passion was to help others through teaching the principles of self-discovery and personal growth. He authored over forty books, including twenty-one New York Times best-sellers. He sadly passed away in 2015 at the age of 75.

Some of the best lessons that I have learned about obtaining happiness and peace, I have learned by listening to the wisdom of Dr. Dyer. He once said that there are no good reasons to worry. He explained that there are only two kinds of situations, the ones we have control over and the ones we don't.

Why should we worry about the things which we have control over? We control the situation, so why worry? Why worry about the things we have no control over? Worrying won't help. Worrying never improves a situation, it just adds stress to it.

Are there some situations, in which our fears or worries are justified? Of course, there are! But, outside of those truly serious occasions, Dr. Dyer makes a valid point. Why spend your time and energy worrying about the small stuff? Making yourself miserable and sick, or losing sleep, isn't going to help in anyway.

When I start to feel stressed out, I try to remember to ask myself if what I'm worried about will affect my life, and my future in the big picture? Will what I'm worried about even matter in five years? If it won't matter in five years, then chances are it probably isn't something worth worrying about today.

FOCUSING ON THE POSITIVE

Have you ever heard of a self-fulfilling prophesy? A self-fulling prophecy is when something happens because we expect it to. In life perception is reality. In other words, the way we think about our lives, has a powerful impact on the quality of our lives. Our perspective is everything.

By placing our focus on the things which we view as being wrong in our lives, we are unconsciously narrowing our perspective, closing ourselves off from happiness, and promoting our own bad experiences. Negative thoughts about ourselves, our situations, or our relationships, tend to spiral downward. As we repeatedly replay these kinds of destructive thoughts in our minds, we become fixed on them and our lives dissolve into a constant state of turmoil, and stress. Every aspect of life becomes tainted. Work, personal relationships, and our health all suffer.

Fortunately, this doesn't have to be the case. Positive thoughts are equally powerful. By consciously choosing to appreciate, enjoy, and be grateful for all that is good in our lives, we can widen the scope of our attention, and multiply our good experiences. When we do that, we become open to the possibilities, we begin to see and appreciate the kindness of others, and we're able to embrace life with a sense of optimism and well-being. This is called being mindful. When we look at the world through this lens, our relationships deepen, we experience more beauty in the world, we become aware of what truly matters in life, we are more kind to ourselves and to others, and good things begin to flow into our lives.

One easy and effective way to help you become more mindful, is to keep a gratitude journal. While this might sound a bit out-there, numerous studies have been done on the effects of positive emotions like gratitude. Researchers have found that gratitude is strongly correlated to, and is an indication of wellbeing. Gratitude has been shown to: improve sleep, improve immune function, benefit the cardiovascular system, lower cortisol in response to stress, reduce the risk of stroke, and to shorten and lesson episodes of depression.

In 2003, the American Psychological Association published the findings from a large research project on gratitude and thankfulness. The project which consisted of three different studies, was conducted by two of the most well-respected experts in the field of phycology, Dr. Robert A. Emmons, and Dr. Michael E. McCullough. Doctors Emmons & McCullough, found that people who kept a gratitude journal were more likely to achieve their goals, felt more optimistic and enthusiastic, and were more likely to help others. One of the studies included a group of people with neuromuscular disease. This group reported: increased levels of energy, better sleep, and feeling more connected to others, after only 21 days of gratitude intervention.

In 2015, a study led by Professor Alex Wood Ph.D. and Dr. Deepak Chopra was also published in the American Psychological Association. The study focused on the effects of gratitude on 186 men and women with asymptomatic Heart Failure. This study found that not only was gratitude associated with: better sleep, less depressed mood, and less fatigue, it was also associated with better self-efficacy, and lower inflammatory biomarkers.

Keeping a gratitude journal takes about 5 minutes out of your day, and will provide you with scientifically proven benefits. Imagine that something as basic as how you view your life, can improve your sleep, your energy, your sense of wellbeing, and can even lower the inflammatory biomarkers in your body!

Here's how to keep a gratitude journal.

1. During the day make a point of noticing the things which make you feel good, appreciative, happy, or that just make you smile.

2. In the evening, find a quite spot where you can sit down and reflect on your day.

3. Write down a few things from your day that you are grateful for. There are no rules as to what you can feel grateful for or as to what you can write down. It can be anything from I am grateful for the sunny weather to I am grateful that my father pulled through his surgery today.

4. Instead of trying to come up with a laundry list of items, take the time to explore and appreciate 2-3 special happenings or people who touched your life in a good way today. Reflect on how they made you feel, why it was special.

5. You can do this exercise every night, 2-3 nights a week, or even just once a week, whichever way works best to you. If you like, keeping your gratitude journal can even become part of your regular bed-time routine.

TAKE FIVE

In today's busy world we are often running, rushing, and under the gun, from early in the morning till we fall into bed at night. Is it any wonder that we can't sleep and we can't seem to relax? To de-stress, we must take breaks from all that hectic craziness. Whether it's in the form of an afternoon walk on your lunch break, taking some time to curl up with a great book and a cup of tea in the evening, meditating, or taking some time to pamper yourself, everyone needs and deserves a little down time to relax and unwind.

FRIENDS, FAMILY, AND COMMUNITY

You've probably heard the saying "it takes a village to raise a child." In part that saying might have evolved from the fact that we need each other, and we're not meant to go it alone. We all need to be part of something bigger than ourselves. We need a community to belong to. In many cultures, though out history, being exiled from your community was the worst possible of punishments because, nothing is as important to our emotional well-being as love, friendship, and community. We all have a need to connect, to be accepted, to be loved.

Today, we create community thorough our loved ones, friends, families, neighbors, religious groups, social groups, and by volunteering. Family game night, date night with your spouse, family gatherings, and going out with your friends is more important than you may have realized. Taking some time to connect with others is a vital part of having a happy, less stressed lifestyle. Personal interactions add meaning, and pleasure to your life. Laughing together with people you care about is good for you, and it's good for them too! It's part of that all-important down time, and it helps create the balance that we all crave, and need.

Our communities not only offer us acceptance and love: they offer us support and understanding. It's good to remember that we're not alone, when we're facing challenges, and it's so rewarding to share good news with someone who's cheering for your success. Make time to spend with those important people in your life. Your life and theirs will be better for it.

Here's a bonus tip, hug someone you love. I know for me; nothing takes the edge off a stressful day better than a tight hug from my husband.

Hugging and cuddling lowers cortisol levels, blood pressure, and reduces stress. One study even found that people who receive more hugs are better protected against catching a cold.

CHAPTER 9

LET'S GET COOKIN'

TIME SAVING COOKING TIPS

You're extremely busy, I get it. I understand what it feels like to work a forty-hour work week while simultaneously trying to take care of your kids, your spouse, your pets, your bills, the grocery shopping, the dentist appointments... The list can go on and on. I can relate because I've been there too, but the best way to control what goes into your body, is to control what goes into your food, and the best way to control what goes into your food, is to make your own meals. To make things easier, I've come up with a few ideas to help you save time in the kitchen.

1. Pick one day a week and prepare 3-4 main meals ahead of time.

2. If you don't want to dedicate an entire day to cooking, cook a day ahead of time. For example: Make a quick grilled or baked salmon dish, serve it with a big veggie filled salad for dinner on Sunday. While you're eating, Monday's chicken can be roasting in the oven. Since Monday's meal is pretty much cooked you can make something which needs a little more prep work, like Super charged chili (in the recipe section), for Tuesday etc. I used this technique many times. Although you're still cooking every day, you're not under so

much pressure to get a decent meal on the table in time for dinner.

3. Always buy and cook extra. By making a big pot of chili, a super large chicken & vegetable stir fry, or extra portions of fish, you get something wonderful, you get leftovers! Leftovers are another great time saver. They make easy hot lunches and quick dinners when time is of the essence or when you just don't feel like fussing, and somehow the food always tastes better the next day.

4. Take tip number 3 a step further, make a huge batch of whatever you decide to cook, portion it off and freeze it for the future. It'll be available to you whenever you need a meal. Just take it out, reheat, and enjoy!

5. Every meal doesn't have to be a culinary master piece! Sometimes going simple is the best way to go. Steak, turkey burgers, lamb chops, or a nice piece of grilled fish, accompanied by a salad and some vegetables, is a quick and easy way to create a delicious meal.

6. Save on clean up time.

   » Use paper plates

   » Cook everything in one pot or pan

   » Cook on the barbeque (at medium – medium low heat)

7. Buy your vegetables already cut up for you. Most grocery store produce departments sell packages of pre-sliced, diced, spiralized, and even riced vegetables, for your convenience. They cost a bit more, but you might find it a valuable time saver. (You can even buy fresh organic garlic that's already been peeled!)

8. Use frozen vegetables, they're just as nutritious as fresh veggies, and they come already cut up for you at less of an expense.

SUGGESTED SHOPPING LIST

Below is a suggested shopping list of some of the staples you'll want to keep on hand.

Dry Goods:	
Nuts & Nut butters	Pumpkin seeds
Sunflower seeds	Flax seeds
Sesame seeds	Caraway seeds
Almond Meal/Flour	Hazelnut flour
Garbanzo bean flour	Coconut flour
Organic 100% raw Cacao powder	Aluminum free baking powder & Soda
Dried parsley	Dried cilantro
Dried dill	Dried rosemary
Garlic powder	Dried basil
Onion powder	Ground cinnamon
Dried turmeric	Ground ginger
Ground cumin	Paprika
Ancho chili powder	Arrow root
Coconut oil	Ghee
Extra virgin olive oil	70 – 88% Cacao chocolate
Organic, full fat canned coconut milk	Mustard powder
Organic, wild, canned salmon	Lentils
Beans	Quinoa (stage 3)
Organic, raw honey (stage 3)	Organic coconut sugar (stage 3)
Organic raw apple cider vinegar	Organic pure vanilla extract
Gluten free soy sauce/Tamari sauce	Canned organic tomato puree
Canned organic crushed tomatoes	Canned organic diced tomatoes
Canned organic whole tomatoes	Canned organic tomato paste
Fresh onions	Fresh garlic
Sweet potatoes	Organic pureed pumpkin
Organic, free range chicken broth	Olives

For the Fridge:	
Pickles in vinegar and salt, not sugar	Sauerkraut
Kimchi	Full fat, organic, grass fed
Greek yogurt	Organic, pastured eggs
Grass fed butter	Bell peppers
Spaghetti squash	Zucchini
Eggplant	Carrots

Celery	Acorn squash
Fresh pumpkin	Fresh berries
Apples	Brussels sprouts
Fresh red cabbage	Peeled organic garlic
Uncured, organic bacon	Fresh salad greens such as: spinach, kale, romaine, and spring mix

For the Freezer:	
Assorted organic frozen vegetables like: spinach, kale, green beans, broccoli, cauliflower, and zucchini	
Frozen berries	Wild fish and shell fish
Ground bison	Grass fed lamb
Grass fed beef	Organic pastured poultry

RECIPES

In this section, my goal is to provide you with a wide variety of tempting recipes that are quick, simple, clear, and as easy to create as possible. Even if you've never cooked before, I want you to enjoy these recipes, and to feel proud to share the food that you make with your friends and family. I've included recipes and tips for meals, sides, baked goods, snacks, desserts, special occasions, and holidays, because being healthy should be inclusive. You deserve to be healthy, and you deserve to have meals that are delightful, tasty, and fun to eat.

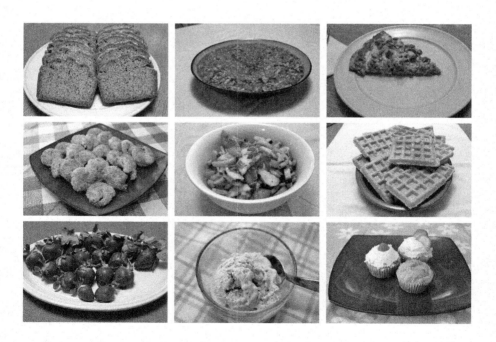

BEVERAGES

In this section, you'll find recipes for homemade coconut milk (an ingredient in many of my recipes), some lovely breakfast shakes, and some of my favorite flavored coffees. Shakes are a good option for people on the go, or for those of you who prefer a lighter breakfast. Both the shakes and the coffee recipes are full of antioxidants, making these beverages a great addition to your morning.

HOMEMADE COCONUT MILK

This coconut milk makes a great dairy replacement in coffee and tea. It's also very useful in cooking, and baking. You'll find that it's called for in many of my recipes.

Yields a little more than 5 ½ cups of coconut milk.

Ingredients:

» One 13.5 ounce can of unsweetened organic coconut milk (make sure the coconut milk is in non-BPA packaging, contains no added sugars, and has as few ingredients as possible).

» 31.5 ounces of filtered water (2-1/3 cans)

DIRECTIONS:

1. Mix one can of unsweetened organic coconut milk with 2 1/3 cans of filtered water.

2. Store in a glass container in the refrigerator.

3. Mix or shake well before using.

HOT COCOA

This beverage isn't meant to be sweet and sugary. Rather, it's meant to be rich and strong, like a cup of black coffee. You can drink it in place of your morning coffee. (Raw cacao is loaded with antioxidants and phytonutrients, it's anti-inflammatory properties make it good for your cardio vascular health, and it's a good source of magnesium too!)

Yield: one serving

Ingredients:

» 1 tbsp. organic raw cacao powder

» ¼ cup homemade coconut milk

» Optional: 1-2 tbsps. pure coconut cream, 1-2 dashes of cinnamon, a drop of mint extract

» About 1 cup filtered hot water

DIRECTIONS:

1. In a large cup or mug, mix the raw cacao powder and coconut milk, until well combined and smooth.

2. Mix in mint extract or cinnamon if desired.

3. Pour in enough hot water to fill the mug.

4. Stir again, and top with coconut cream (and more cinnamon,) if you wish.

5. Enjoy with breakfast, or anytime.

MOCHA LATTE

Yield: one serving

Ingredients:

» 1 tbsp. organic raw cacao powder

» ¼ homemade coconut milk

» 1-2 Tbsps. pure coconut cream

» 1 dash of cinnamon

» About 1 cup hot coffee

DIRECTIONS:

1. In a large cup or mug, mix the raw cacao powder, and coconut milk, until well combined and smooth.

2. Pour in enough hot coffee to fill the mug, and stir gently.

3. Top with coconut cream and a dash of cinnamon.

4. Enjoy with breakfast, or have it later in the day for dessert.

DARK CHOCOLATE FLAVORED COFFEE

Yield: 12 servings

Ingredients:

- » 2 tbsp. organic raw cacao powder
- » Enough coffee to make a 12-cup pot of coffee

DIRECTIONS:

1. Set up your coffee machine to brew a 12-cup pot of coffee.
2. Place 2 tbsps. of organic raw cacao powder on top of the coffee in the coffee filter, and brew as usual.

CHOCOLATE CHAI FLAVORED COFFEE

Yield: 12 servings

Ingredients:

- » 1 1/2 tbsps. organic raw cacao powder
- » ¼ tsp ground cinnamon
- » ¼ tsp. ground ginger
- » 1/8 tsp. ground cardamom
- » 1/8 tsp. ground cloves
- » Enough coffee to make a 12-cup pot of coffee

DIRECTIONS:

1. Set up your coffee machine to brew a 12-cup pot of coffee.
2. Place the organic raw cacao powder and the spices, on top of the coffee in the coffee filter, and brew as usual.

CHOCOLATE MINT FLAVORED COFFEE

Yield: 12 servings

Ingredients:

- » 1 1/2 tbsps. organic raw cacao powder
- » 1 tbsp. dried mint

DIRECTIONS:

1. Set up your coffee machine to brew a 12-cup pot of coffee.

2. Place the organic raw cacao powder and the mint on top of the coffee in the coffee filter, and brew as usual.

CHOCOLATE SNICKERDOODLE FLAVORED COFFEE

Yield: 12 servings

Ingredients:

» 1 1/2 tbsps. organic raw cacao powder

» ½ tsp ground cinnamon

» ¼ tsp. ground ginger

» 1/8 tsp. ground cardamom

» Enough coffee to make a 12-cup pot of coffee

DIRECTIONS:

1. Set up your coffee machine to brew a 12-cup pot of coffee.

2. Place the organic raw cacao powder and the spices on top of the coffee in the coffee filter, and brew as usual.

GINGERBREAD FLAVORED COFFEE

Yield: 12 servings

Ingredients:

» ¼ tsp. ground ginger

» ¼ tsp. ground cinnamon

» Enough coffee to make a 12-cup pot of coffee

DIRECTIONS:

1. Set up your coffee machine to brew a 12-cup pot of coffee.

2. Place the spices on top of the coffee in the coffee filter, and brew as usual.

BANANA BERRY SHAKE

This shake makes a delicious breakfast for those days when you're short on time. You can have an additional protein with it if you're very hungry, but you don't have to, because the almonds give you a healthy dose of good fat and protein.

Yields one serving

Ingredients:

- » 1/8 cup almonds
- » 1 cup homemade coconut milk
- » ½ cup fresh raspberries and blackberries
- » 1/3 frozen banana
- » 4 red grapes
- » 3 ice cubes
- » 2-3 dashes of cinnamon
- » 1-2 drops of pure vanilla extract

DIRECTIONS:

1. Place all the ingredients into a high-powered blender.
2. Blend until smooth.

SUPER CHARGED SHAKE

This shake will start your day off with plenty of phytonutrients, your daily dose of selenium, and a focused mind! (To avoid stomach upset, if you have never used MCT oil before, or if you're not yet accustomed to larger quantities of MCT oil, you can use less or substitute it with some coconut oil.) This beverage doesn't have much protein, so you'll either have to eat some protein on the side, or you can add a scoop of a quality protein powder to the shake.

Yields one serving

Ingredients:

- » 1 cup of greens
- » 1 cup of frozen mixed berries
- » 2 brazil nuts
- » 1 1/8 cups homemade coconut milk
- » 1 Tbsp. of MCT oil or coconut oil
- » 2-3 ice cubes

DIRECTIONS:

1. Place all the ingredients into a high-powered blender.
2. Blend until smooth.

FALL HARVEST SHAKE

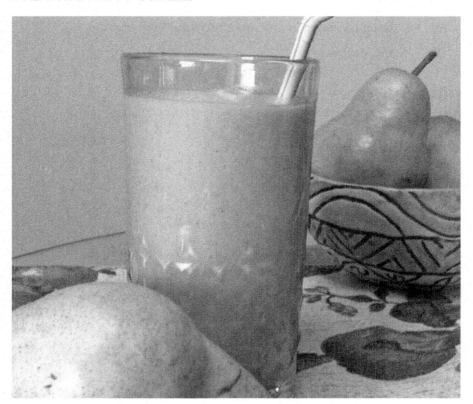

Yield: 2 servings

Ingredients:

- » 1 fresh pear
- » ½ cup of cooked pumpkin
- » ¼ cup almonds
- » 4 dashes of cinnamon
- » ½ x ½" piece of fresh ginger, peeled
- » 2 pinches of nutmeg
- » 2 pinches of allspice
- » 2 cups of homemade coconut milk
- » 4 ice cubes

DIRECTIONS:

1. Place all the ingredients into a high-powered blender.
2. Blend until smooth.

PB&J SHAKE

This one is my favorite shake so far.

Yields one serving

Ingredients:

- » 1 cup of berries
- » 2 tbsp. organic, all natural, peanut butter
- » 1 cup homemade coconut milk

DIRECTIONS:

1. Place all the ingredients into a high-powered blender.
2. Blend until smooth.

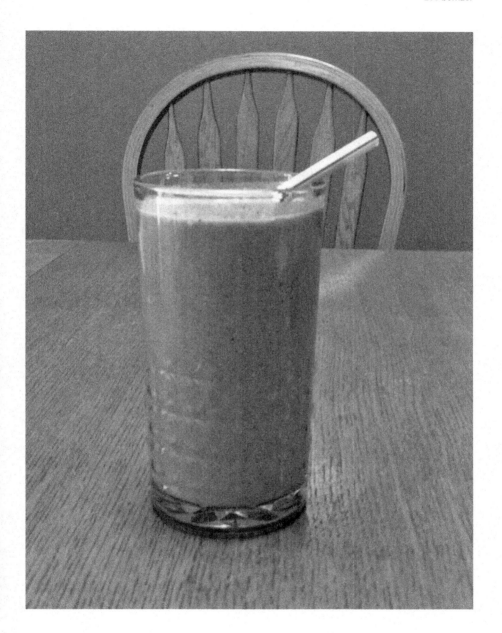

BREAKFAST

Breakfast is many things to many people. Below, I've given you a few basic breakfast recipes, but there are no rules. You can eat whatever you want to for breakfast. Whether it be a quick shake, a fresh omelet that's loaded with veggies, or last night's leftovers, it's completely up to you! You might also create your own recipes, or use recipes from other parts of the book to make the breakfast that suits you best. I'd also like to remind you that if you're not hungry, you shouldn't eat breakfast until you are. Don't let a clock on the wall tell you when to eat, let your own body be your guide.

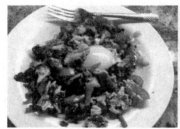 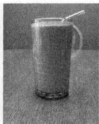 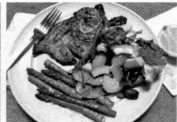

FULL-FAT DAIRY GREEK YOGURT

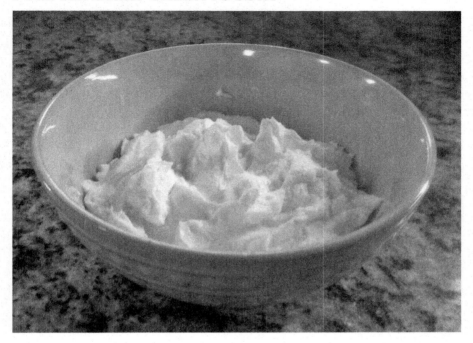

I have found it surprisingly difficult to find full fat, grass fed, organic Greek yogurt, but you can turn your favorite brand of regular yogurt into Greek yogurt by following a few easy steps.

1. Place 2 large coffee filters inside a strainer.

2. Place the strainer over a large bowl.

3. Spoon the yogurt of your choice into the strainer.

4. Place the strainer and bowl in the refrigerator for about 4 hours, or until it is thickened to your liking.

5. Store your Greek yogurt in the refrigerator in a covered container.

The result is a thick, creamy yogurt, with as much protein as store-bought Greek yogurt.

NON-DAIRY COCONUT MILK YOGURT

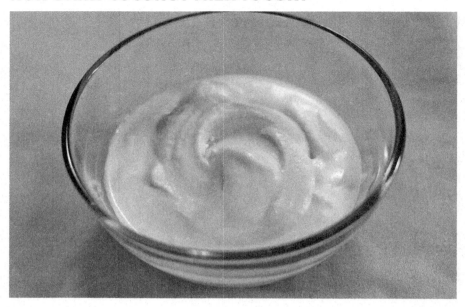

This yogurt is a good dairy free option for those of you who are lactose intolerant, and for those who are trying to avoid dairy. Remember though, that coconut milk yogurt does not contain the protein normally found dairy yogurt, and adjust your meal accordingly.

Yield: 27 oz.

Ingredients:

» 2 cans organic coconut milk

» 2 probiotic capsules, with about 30 billion live cultures per capsule. (For the best results, be sure the probiotic you're using contains lactobacillus, acidophilous, or S. thermophiles. A combination works best.)

DIRECTIONS:

1. Choose a large glass jar with a lid, or a large glass dish with a lid, for your yogurt container.

2. Sterilize your container and its lid. You can use your dishwasher to sterilize your container and lid, or do the following: 1st Place a metal spoon into your chosen glass container, and carefully fill it with boiling water. 2nd Place the lid on tightly. 3rd Wrap a towel around the covered container. Very carefully and gently, shake the container (away from your face and over a sink) to ensure the lid also gets sterilized. 4th Uncover the container, drain out the water and set on the side to cool.

3. When you open the cans of coconut milk, you will notice that it has separated into coconut cream on the top, and coconut water on the bottom. Scoop the coconut cream into a clean bowl, and use a fork to gently beat it until it's smooth.

4. Mix the remaining liquid into the coconut cream a little bit at a time, until it is fully incorporated.

5. Open the probiotic capsules and empty the contents into the coconut milk. Mix to combine.

6. Pour the yogurt into your glass container, and tightly cover it with its lid.

7. Turn on the oven light.

8. Place the container into the oven close to the oven light, and cover it with a dish towel. The oven light should keep the temperature inside the oven at about 110 F, which is the correct temperature to incubate yogurt at.

9. Leave the yogurt in the oven for 18-24 hours.

10. Unwrap the yogurt, and place it in the refrigerator to chill overnight or for about 12 hours. It will thicken slightly as it chills. When the yogurt is completely chilled, you will have a thin yogurt that is similar in thickness to kefir.

11. To thicken the yogurt place 2 coffee filters into a large mesh strainer, and place the strainer over a large bowl. Pour the yogurt

into the filters, and place the bowl with the strainer into the refrigerator to chill for 3-4 hours, or until the yogurt has reached the desired thickness.

You can eat this yogurt with some berries on top, use it in a smoothie, or serve it with something spicy as a pallet cleanser. This yogurt will get even better in a day or two, if it lasts that long!

FLUFFY ALMOND FLOUR PANCAKES

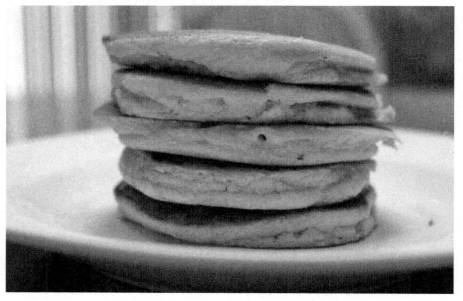

These pancakes have the same texture as the pancakes that most of us grew up with. They taste great, are easy to make, and every bite is a mouthful of happiness!

Yield: 15 pancakes

Serving size: 3 pancakes

Ingredients:

» 2 cups almond meal/flour

» 1 tsp baking soda

- » 1 pinch of sea salt
- » 1 dash of ground cinnamon
- » 2 large eggs
- » 2 large egg whites
- » 3/4 tsp pure vanilla extract
- » approx. 1/2 cup water
- » 1-2 tsp of extra virgin coconut oil, or grass-fed butter

DIRECTIONS:

1. In a medium bowl, use a whisk to combine the dry ingredients.

2. In a separate bowl, use a whisk to combine the eggs and the vanilla.

3. Stir the dry ingredients into the egg mixture, and stir in enough water to make the batter the same consistency as regular pancake batter.

4. Melt your oil in a non-stick pan or griddle that is heated to about 350° F.

5. Pour large spoons of pancake batter onto the griddle.

6. Cook until edges are dry and bubbles appear on the tops. Flip the pancakes over, and cook until cooked through and golden on both sides.

7. Serve with eggs, uncured bacon or ham, and fresh fruit, nut butter, or Raw Raspberry Sauce (find the recipe in the breakfast section).

GRAIN FREE PUMPKIN PANCAKES

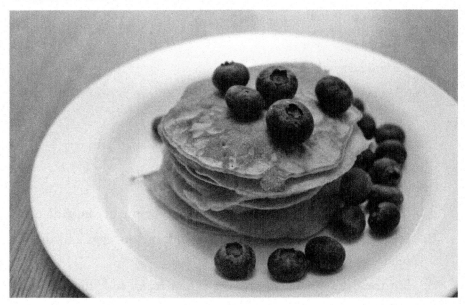

These delicate little pancakes are a delightful treat for breakfast. They combine the wholesome goodness of pumpkin with the comforting flavors of cinnamon and ginger.

Yield: approx. 21 small pancakes

Serving size: 7 pancakes

Ingredients:

- » 1 cup pureed pumpkin
- » 3 large eggs
- » 2 large egg whites
- » 1/4 cup almond meal/flour
- » 3/4 tsp ground cinnamon
- » 1/2 tsp ground ginger
- » 1/8 tsp. allspice
- » a pinch of salt
- » 1-2 tsp of extra virgin coconut oil, or grass-fed butter

DIRECTIONS:

1. Place all the ingredients, except oil/butter, into the blender.

2. Blend until well combined. For the last few seconds, put the blender on whip to aerate the batter.

3. Melt your oil in a non-stick pan or griddle that is heated to about 350° F.

4. Pour small amounts of pancake batter onto the griddle.

5. Cook until bubbles cover the top. Flip the pancakes over, and cook until cooked through and golden on both sides.

6. Serve with eggs, uncured bacon, or ham, and fresh fruit, nut butter, or Raw Raspberry Sauce (found in this section).

WAFFLES

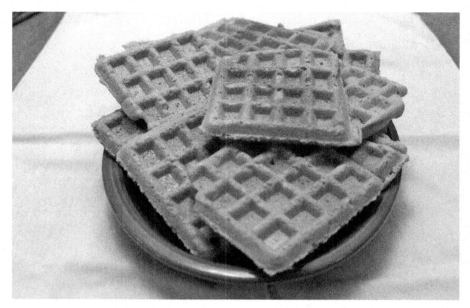

These waffles may be the best you've ever tasted. They're thick, crispy on the outside, and tender on the inside. They freeze well, and can be toasted straight from the freezer. Once you've had them, they'll be the only waffles for you!

Yield: 16 waffles

Ingredients:

- » 4 cups almond meal/flour
- » 2 tsp baking soda
- » 2 pinches of sea salt
- » 2 dashes of ground cinnamon
- » 4 large eggs
- » 4 large egg whites
- » 2 tsp pure vanilla extract
- » 1 3/4 cup homemade coconut milk (recipe in this section)

DIRECTIONS:

1. In a medium bowl, use a whisk to combine the dry ingredients.

2. In a separate bowl, use a whisk to combine the eggs, vanilla, and coconut milk.

3. Whisk the dry ingredients into the egg mixture.

4. Preheat a waffle iron, and spray liberally with cooking spray.

5. Pour about ¼ cup of batter for each waffle, onto the cooking surface of the waffle iron.

6. Cook per manufacturer's instructions, or for approximately 5 minutes until there is no longer steam coming from the waffle iron.

7. Repeat steps 4-6, until you run out of batter.

8. Serve immediately. Store leftovers in an airtight container in the freezer.

RAW RASPBERRY SAUCE

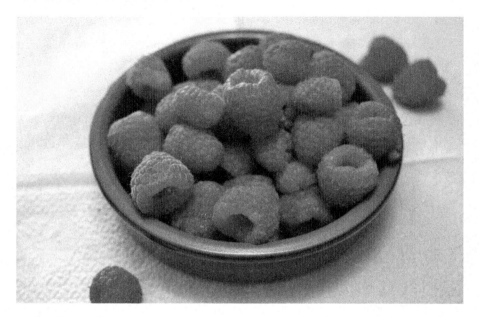

Fresh raspberries in season are so outstandingly sweet, they make a perfect sauce for topping pancakes or waffles. To make this sauce is so simple; it's more of a tip than a recipe.

Just place a cup or two of fresh, organic raspberries into the blender, add just enough water to process them, and blend into a sauce. That's it! In seconds, you'll have a fresh raspberry pancake topping.

BREAKFAST QUINOA – STAGE 3 ONLY

Here's a gluten-free hot breakfast cereal that I developed for my husband. Serving to serving, it's got 3 times more protein and twice as much fiber as a bowl of steel cut oats. It also contains a good amount of calcium, potassium, and iron. You can make it ahead, and serve it warm or cold for a convenient and filling breakfast on the go.

Yield: 6 servings

Serving size: 1/2 cup

Added sugar per serving: ½ tsp.

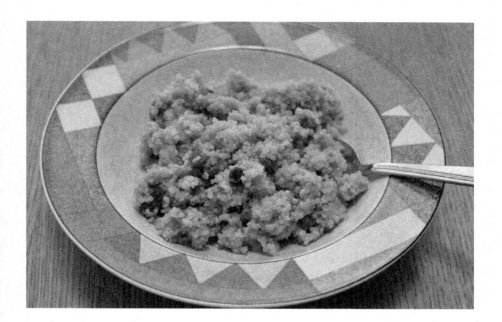

Ingredients:

- » 1 1/2 cups organic quinoa, rinsed
- » 3 cups unsweetened, homemade coconut milk (see recipe)
- » 1 tbsp. organic coconut sugar, raw honey, or pure maple syrup
- » A pinch of salt
- » organic cinnamon to taste
- » up to 6 tbsp. of optional stir-ins such as: 2 tbsps. organic raisins or other organic dried fruit, chopped nuts, organic unsweetened coconut flakes, hulled pumpkin seeds, hulled sunflower seeds, or flax seeds.

DIRECTIONS:

1. Place all the ingredients into a medium saucepan, and place it on the stove top.
2. Over medium-high heat, mixing occasionally, bring the contents of the saucepan to a boil.

3. Lower the heat to the lowest possible setting. Cover the pan, and allow to simmer for about 15 minutes, until all the liquid has been absorbed.

4. Remove the mixture from the heat, and fluff it with a fork. Place the lid back on the pan, and allow it to rest for another 15 minutes.

5. Uncover the quinoa, and fluff it once more. It's now ready to be eaten.

Once it has cooled, you can store it covered, in the refrigerator. You can even portion it out ahead of time, for convenience. In addition to the stir-ins, you might also enjoy topping your Breakfast Quinoa with a pat of grass fed butter, or a spoonful of organic extra virgin coconut oil. If you like, you can forego the stir-ins at the beginning of the recipe, and mix some fresh fruit, nuts, or nut butters right into your bowl. Experiment and enjoy it your favorite way.

PUMPKIN CHEESE BLINTZ CASSEROLE – STAGE 3 ONLY

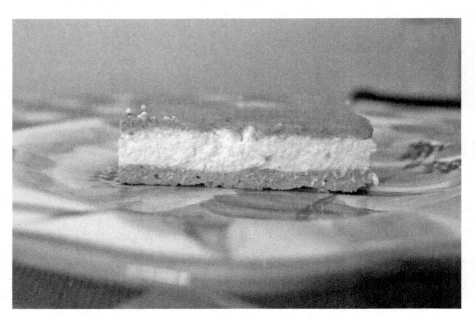

This dish is perfect as part of a holiday brunch or luncheon.

Yield: 12 squares

Serving size: 1 square

Added sugar per serving: ½ tsp.

Ingredients for pumpkin batter:

- » 2 cup pureed pumpkin
- » 6 large eggs
- » 4 large egg whites
- » 1/2 cup almond meal/flour
- » 1 1/2 tsp ground cinnamon
- » 1 tsp ground ginger
- » 1/4 tsp. allspice
- » 2 pinches of salt

Ingredients for cheese filling:

- » 3 cups ricotta
- » 4 oz. cream cheese, softened
- » 2 large pastured eggs
- » 1 tbsp. fresh lemon juice
- » ½ tsp. pure vanilla extract
- » 2 tbsp. organic raw honey

DIRECTIONS:

1. Preheat the oven to 350° F.

2. Grease the bottom and sides of a 9x13 baking pan with coconut oil or butter.

3. Place all the ingredients for the batter, into the bowl of a food

processor that has been fitted with a steel blade.

4. Process until the batter is well combined and smooth.

5. In a large bowl, combine the ingredients for the filling. Mix well with a fork, until the filling is evenly combined.

6. Pour 1 ½ cups of the batter into the prepared pan. Spread the batter with the back of a spoon to make sure it is evenly distributed, and covers the bottom of the pan.

7. Place the pan onto the center rack of the preheated oven, and bake for approximately 15 minutes until it is set.

8. Remove the pan from the oven. Spread the cheese filling evenly over the bottom crust.

9. Return to the oven, and bake for another 30 minutes.

10. Remove the pan from the oven. Spread the remaining pumpkin batter over the top of the filling. Return the pan to the oven, and bake for another 15-20 minutes, until the top layer is baked.

11. Let cool for 10-15 minutes before slicing.

12. Cut the casserole into 12 squares.

CHEESY MUSHROOM AND KALE QUICHE

This Cheesy Mushroom and Kale Quiche is so gooey, rich, and delectable. It's packed with protein, and contains Vitamin A, Vitamin C, potassium, calcium, and iron. Enjoy a double serving with some fresh berries for that special breakfast, or serve your guests a slice with a big healthy salad for lunch.

To make a more traditional quiche for a decadent side dish or appetizer, simply use heavy cream instead of cottage cheese in this recipe.

Yield: 8 servings

Ingredients:

» 10 ounces frozen chopped kale

- » 8 white mushrooms, sliced
- » 1/4 cup minced onion
- » 1 glove of garlic, minced
- » 4 large organic, pastured eggs
- » 1/4 lb. thinly sliced, organic Swiss cheese
- » 1 1/2 cups organic full fat cottage cheese
- » black pepper to taste
- » paprika to taste
- » dried cilantro for the top
- » dried dill for the top

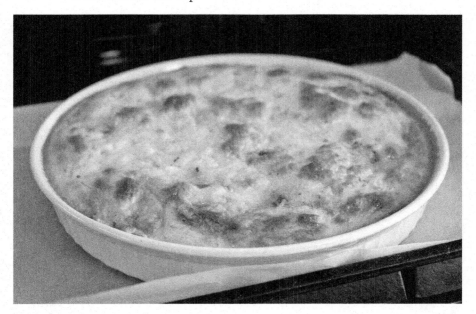

DIRECTIONS:

1. Preheat the oven to 375 F.
2. Grease a 10" quiche dish.
3. Thaw the kale in the microwave, and carefully squeeze out any extra water.
4. Spread the kale evenly in the bottom of the quiche dish. Layer all

of the mushrooms evenly over the kale.

5. Layer all the cheese evenly over the mushrooms, and press the mixture down with your hands.

6. In a large bowl, gently mix the eggs, onion, garlic, paprika, and black pepper.

7. Carefully fold in the cottage cheese.

8. Pour the egg mixture evenly over the rest of the quiche.

9. Generously sprinkle some cilantro and dill over the top.

10. Place the quiche on the center rack of the preheated oven, and cook for about 35-40 minutes, or until the top is golden brown and the filling is set.

11. Let cool for a few minutes before serving. Leftovers can be stored covered in the refrigerator, after it is fully cooled off. Like many good dishes, this quiche is even better the next day.

BROCCOLI CHEDDAR QUICHE

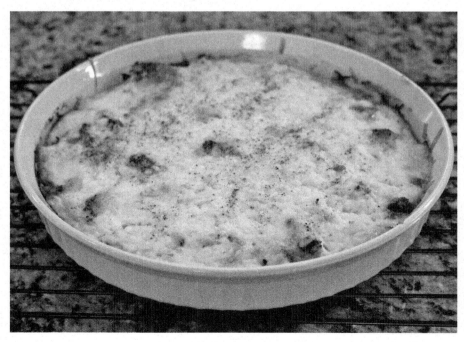

My daughter told me she likes this dish so much, that she could easily see it satisfying a craving for mac n cheese!

To make a more traditional quiche for a decadent side dish or appetizer, simply use heavy cream instead of cottage cheese in this recipe.

Yield: 8 servings

Ingredients:

- » 12 ounces of frozen organic broccoli florets, thawed and drained
- » 4 ounces of organic cheddar cheese, shredded
- » 4 large organic, pastured eggs
- » 1 1/2 cups organic, full fat cottage cheese
- » 1/4 tsp sea salt
- » 1/8 tsp mustard powder
- » black pepper to taste
- » paprika to taste

DIRECTIONS:

1. Preheat the oven to 375 F.
2. Grease a 10" quiche dish.
3. Spread the broccoli evenly on the bottom of the quiche dish.
4. Layer all the cheese evenly over the broccoli.
5. In a large bowl, gently mix the eggs, salt, pepper, mustard powder, and paprika.
6. Carefully fold in the cottage cheese.
7. Pour the egg mixture evenly over the rest of the quiche.
8. Evenly sprinkle some more paprika over the top.
9. Place the quiche on the center rack of the preheated oven, and cook for about 35-40 minutes, or until the top is golden brown and the filling is set.

10. Let cool for a few minutes before serving. Leftovers can be stored covered in the refrigerator, after it is fully cooled.

SALADS, SOUPS, AND STEWS

FRESH CUCUMBER AND TOMATO SALAD

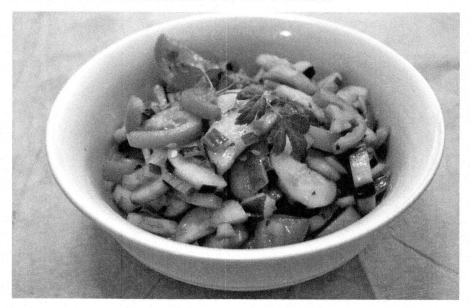

This salad is refreshing, and has a bright, crisp flavor.

Yield: 6 cups

Serving size: 1/2 cup

Ingredients:

- » 1/2 cup balsamic vinegar
- » 1 tsp fresh oregano
- » 1 tsp fresh parsley
- » 2/3 tsp fresh thyme
- » 1 clove of garlic
- » 1/4 tsp sea salt
- » 1/8 tsp black pepper
- » 2/3 cup extra virgin olive oil
- » 2 cucumbers, peeled, sliced into rounds, and cut in half
- » 6 Roma tomatoes, sliced into rounds and cut in half

» 3/4 cup red onion, diced

» extra salt and pepper, optional

DIRECTIONS:

1. Place the first seven ingredients into the bowl of a food processor that has been fitted with a steel blade.

2. Begin blending. While the processor is running, slowly pour the olive oil through the feed tube, into the bowl.

3. Blend for a few seconds, until the dressing is thoroughly combined and becomes opaque.

4. Place the cucumbers, tomatoes, and onion into a large bowl.

5. Pour the dressing into the bowl, and mix well to combine all the ingredients.

6. Add more salt and pepper to taste, if desired.

7. Chill salad in a covered container in the refrigerator, for at least 4 hours, to allow the flavors to meld before serving.

FOOD BOWLS

Food bowls are like creative salads. You can put anything you like into them, and you can use whatever you have on hand. For example, you can top leftover spaghetti squash with chopped apples, chicken, bacon, walnuts, and pumpkin seeds; or you can top grape tomatoes, cucumber chunks, avocado slices, chopped celery, and shredded carrots with a can of wild salmon. Another great idea is to chop up everything you that would have in your favorite sandwich, and toss it into a bowl. My daughter's favorite is turkey, avocado, tomatoes, bacon, and HBC mayo. (You can find the recipe for the mayonnaise in the condiments section.) You can even use cold leftover veggies and last night's protein to make a food bowl. They're fun to eat, and they're way better then any chain restaurant food bowl.

One of my favorite food bowls is a combination of cold leftover veggies like broccoli and cauliflower, with leftover chicken or pork. I add a little coconut milk, a spoonful or two of almond butter and peanut butter, and a couple of dashes of hot sauce. Then, I warm it in the microwave. When it's warm, I mix it and top it with some chopped nuts or some pumpkin seeds. I love it because it reminds me of Tai food, and it's so easy to throw together. These also make great lunches for work days. Just toss together a food bowl the night before, and store it in a glass container in the fridge overnight. In the morning, just grab and go.

NY STYLE COLE SLAW – STAGE 3 ONLY

What can I say, except my family and I just love this slaw! It goes with everything, and I think it beats store bought on any day of the week. For the best flavor, make it a day ahead.

Yield: 8 servings

Serving size: ½ cup

Added sugar per serving: about 1/3 tsp.

Ingredients:

- » 1 lb. coleslaw mix (shredded cabbage and carrots)
- » 1/3 cup white vinegar
- » 1/3 cup filtered water
- » 1 tbsp. organic coconut sugar
- » 2/3 cup HBC Mayo (find recipe under condiments)
- » ½ tsp. celery seed
- » ½ tsp onion powder
- » Iodized sea salt and black pepper to taste

DIRECTIONS:

1. Place the coleslaw mix into a large bowl and set aside.
2. In a separate bowl, combine the vinegar, water, sugar, mayo, celery seed, and onion powder. Mix well to make the dressing.
3. Pour the dressing over the slaw mix. Mix and massage the salad with your hands, to release the juices from the cabbage, and to tenderize your coleslaw.
4. Cover and refrigerate overnight to allow the flavors to meld, and cabbage to cure.

BROCCOLI SALAD – STAGE 3 ONLY

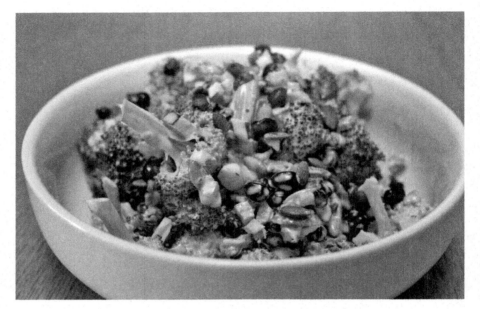

This broccoli salad is a gourmet dish that you can feel proud to serve at the next family picnic or potluck dinner. You can double the recipe if you're feeding a large crowd.

Yield: 4 cups

Serving size: 1 cup

Added sugar per serving: about 1/3 tsp.

Ingredients:

> » ¾ lb. fresh broccoli florets
> » ¼ of a red onion, minced
> » 1 tbsp. hulled pumpkin or sunflower seeds
> » 2 pieces of uncured bacon, cooked and crumbled
> » ¼ cup pomegranate arils

Dressing Ingredients:

> » 2/3 cup HBC Mayo (find recipe under condiments)
> » 1 tbsp. filtered water

» 1 tbsp. organic white vinegar

» 1/4 tsp celery seed

» 1 ½ tsp. raw honey

DIRECTIONS:

1. In a small bowl, combine all the ingredients for the dressing. Mix well, and set on the side.

2. Place all the remaining ingredients into a large bowl, and toss well.

3. Pour the dressing over the salad, and toss again.

4. Garnish with a few additional pomegranate arils if desired.

5. Refrigerate for several hours or overnight, to allow the flavors to meld.

LEMONY QUINOA SALAD – STAGE 3 ONLY

Delicious as a side, this salad easily transitions into a nice dinner. Add in some cooked chicken or shellfish, and voilà! A simple, and flavorful, light summer meal is ready to go!

Yield: 4 cups

Serving size: 1/2 cup

Ingredients:

» 1 cup of plain quinoa

» 2 cups of organic free-range chicken broth

» 1 cup of frozen peas & carrots

» 1 Tbsp. fresh lemon juice

» 2 Tbsp. red onion, minced

» 2/3 cup quinoa salad dressing (recipe included below)

DIRECTIONS:

1. In a 2qt sauce pan, bring the broth to a boil. Mix in the quinoa, and the peas & carrots, and cover.

2. Lower heat all the way down to low. Simmer covered, until the quinoa is tender, and all the liquid has been absorbed.

3. Place the mixture into a large bowl, and set aside to cool.

4. While the quinoa is cooling, prepare the dressing as per the recipe.

5. When the dressing is ready, stir 2/3 a cup of the dressing into the quinoa.

6. Mix in the lemon juice and the red onions.

7. Place the salad, uncovered, on an open rack in the refrigerator, to chill.

8. Once the salad is chilled, you can serve it, or cover it and serve it later.

QUINOA SALAD DRESSING

Yield: 1 cup

Ingredients:

- » 1/3 cup apple cider vinegar
- » 2/3 cup extra virgin olive oil
- » 1 clove of garlic
- » 1 tsp fresh oregano
- » 1 tsp fresh parsley
- » 1/2 tsp sea salt
- » 1/8 tsp black pepper
- » 1/4 tsp celery seed
- » 1/8 tsp. ground coriander seed

DIRECTIONS:

1. Place all the ingredients, except for the olive oil, into the bowl of a food processor that has been fitted with a steel blade.

2. Begin blending. While the processor is running, slowly pour the olive oil through the feed tube into the bowl.

3. Blend for a few seconds, until the dressing is thoroughly combined and becomes opaque.

LEAFLESS CHOPPED SALAD

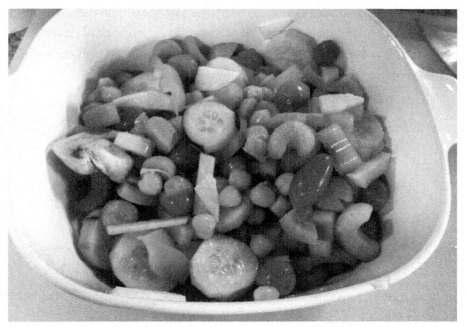

This salad is a lot like a giant version of the food bowl; it's meant to feed a small group of people as an alternative to a traditional salad. It's perfect for those times when you want a break from the usual, and it's a great way to get in a nice variety of rainbow colors into your meal. As with the food bowls, the sky's the limit when it comes to creating the perfect salad. The one pictured above has orange bell peppers, cucumber, mushrooms, jicama, celery, olives, grape tomatoes, and chickpeas, but you can make yours using anything that you have on hand, or that you would enjoy. Here's a list of possible ingredients to consider when building your salad: shredded raw asparagus, radishes, avocado, bell peppers, beets, artichokes, chopped cucumber or zucchini, mushrooms, raw carrots, spiralized raw sweet potato, celery, cooked beans, tomatoes, jicama, fresh broccoli or cauliflower florets, fresh green beans, sugar snap peas, sprouts, fresh herbs, onions, olives, shredded red cabbage, apples, berries, cranberries, orange chunks, nuts, and seeds.

CHICKEN FAJITA SOUP

This hardy soup makes a wonderful one pot meal. Have it for supper one night, and for lunch the next day. It would be wonderful served with some fresh rye bread, biscuits, or snack crackers. (You can find the recipes for these items in the baking section of this book.)

Yields 4-8 large bowls of soup

Ingredients:

- » 5 split chicken breasts, rinsed
- » 2 carrots, washed, peeled, and sliced into rounds
- » 2 stalks of celery, washed, and sliced
- » 10 oz. frozen spinach
- » 1 onion, diced
- » 1 bell red pepper, washed, seeded, and diced
- » 28 oz. can crushed tomatoes
- » 15 oz. can chickpeas, rinsed and drained
- » 4 cloves of garlic, minced
- » 1 1/2 tbsp. paprika
- » 3/4 tsp cumin
- » 3/4 tsp ancho chili powder
- » 2 tsp dried cilantro
- » 1/2 tsp dried oregano
- » 1/2 tsp turmeric powder
- » 2 tbsp. store bought salsa verde (look for one with no added sugar)
- » Filtered water

» Iodized sea salt & black pepper

» 1 avocado for the garnish

DIRECTIONS:

1. Place the chicken breasts in the bottom of an 8qt soup pot.

2. Keep the canned tomatoes and the salsa on the side for later use. Place all the remaining vegetables, the beans, and the spices on top of the chicken in the pot.

3. Fill the pot with water to cover the soup ingredients. The water level should be only about 2-3" below the top of the pot.

4. Place the pot on the stove, and bring to a full boil over a medium-high heat.

5. When the soup comes to a full boil, lower the heat. You want the soup to be cooking at a slow, gentle boil. If the soup is bubbling over the top of the pot, you need to lower the heat a bit more.

6. Continue to cook uncovered, for about an hour.

7. After about an hour, mix your soup, using a large metal spoon. Check the chicken with a fork to see if it is cooked through and tender.

8. When the chicken is tender, remove it from the pot and place it in a large dish. Set the dish on the side, for now.

9. Add the tomatoes and the salsa to the soup. Mix well, and add salt and pepper to taste.

10. To serve, shred some chicken into a bowl, top with heaping spoonfuls of the vegetables, and ladle some broth over the top. Garnish each bowl with chunks of fresh avocado.

GREEN GOODNESS SOUP

This quick, nourishing soup makes a great accompaniment to any meal. It also makes a nice afternoon snack.

Yield: 1-2 servings

Ingredients:

- » 1 cup fresh or frozen spinach
- » 1 cup homemade coconut milk (see recipe)
- » ½ cup organic free-range chicken broth
- » The juice of one lemon wedge
- » ½ a leek, washed and dried
- » 1 clove of raw garlic
- » 1 tbsp. of dried dill
- » Salt and pepper
- » Olive oil

DIRECTIONS:

1. Place all the ingredients except the salt, pepper, and olive oil, into a high-speed blender with a soup setting.
2. Blend on soup setting, until done.
3. Add salt and pepper to taste and pour into bowls.
4. Garnish with a drizzle of olive oil.
5. If your blender doesn't have a soup setting, blend until smooth, and warm on the stove or in the microwave.

SPICY GREEN SOUP

Here's another quick soup recipe.

Yield: 1-2 servings

Ingredients:

- » 2 cups of greens
- » 2 tbsp. walnuts
- » 2 cups of organic free-range chicken broth
- » 1 clove of raw garlic

- » ¼ tsp. cumin
- » ¼ cup store bought salsa verde (look for one with no added sugar)
- » Cream cheese

DIRECTIONS:

1. Place all the ingredients, except the cream cheese, into a high-speed blender with a soup setting.
2. Blend on soup setting until done, and pour into bowls.
3. Garnish with bits of cream cheese.
4. If your blender doesn't have a soup setting, blend until smooth, and warm on the stove or in the microwave.

LAMB RAGOUT SOUP

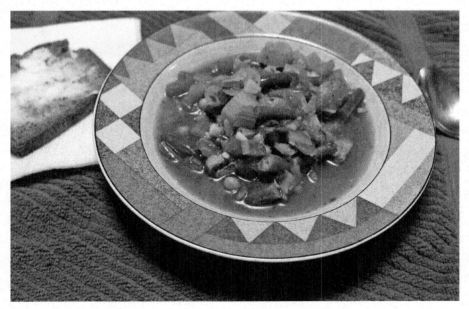

This soup was sort of a happy accident. You see, I wanted to make a soup out of beef bone broth, but I couldn't find any bone in, grass-fed beef at my local supermarket. I decided to buy some grass-fed lamb chops instead. My family loved the resulting soup so much that I decided to share the recipe with you. I served it for the first time as dinner on a chilly December night. A piece of rustic bread (find recipe in the baking section), slathered with some grass-fed butter was the perfect final addition to this very hearty meal.

This soup is best made early in the day, or the day before. It needs to be refrigerated for enough hours to allow the excess lamb fat to rise to the top, so that it can be removed from the soup. This is done so that the finished soup will rich, but not too greasy.

Yield: 4 quarts of soup

Ingredients:

» 2 lb. center cut, bone in, lamb chops

» ¾ cup organic peas (stage 3 only, omit for stage 2)

» 6 stalks of celery, washed, and sliced, into ¼" pieces

» 3 fresh carrots; washed, peeled, and sliced into ¼" rounds

» 1 large onion; washed, peeled, and chopped

» 5 cloves of garlic, peeled and chopped

» 2 tsp. dried parsley

» 1 tsp. dried thyme

» ¼ tsp. dried oregano

» 1 tsp. turmeric powder

» ¼ tsp. cumin powder

» Salt & pepper

» Filtered water

» 28 oz. can of organic diced tomatoes

» 12-16 oz. of cooked vegetables such as, broccoli, cauliflower, green beans, or brussels sprouts. (A good way to make use of leftover vegetables.)

DIRECTIONS:

1. Place lamb chops into the bottom of an 8-quart soup pot.

2. Keeping the tomatoes and the cooked vegetables on the side for now, place the other vegetables, and the measured spices on top of the lamb.

3. Fill the pot 2/3 of the way up with water.

4. Place the pot on the stove, and bring to a full boil over a medium-high heat.

5. When the soup comes to a full boil, lower the heat. You want the soup to be cooking at a slow, gentle boil. If the soup is bubbling over the top of the pot, you need to lower the heat a bit more.

6. Continue to cook uncovered for about an hour.

7. After about an hour, mix your soup using a large metal spoon. Check the lamb with a fork to see if it is cooked through and tender.

8. When the meat is tender, remove it from the pot and place it in a large dish. Set the dish on the side to cool.

9. Add the tomatoes, and the cooked vegetables to the soup. Mix well, and add salt and pepper to taste.

10. Cook for 10 more minutes.

11. When the soup is done, set it on a cooling rack to cool for a while. (For food safety, don't leave the soup on the counter for more than 2 hours.)

12. While the soup is cooling, remove the lamb from the bone, and cut it into cubes.

13. Place the cubed lamb into a sealed container, and put into the fridge for now.

14. When the soup is no longer boiling hot, place it uncovered on an open rack in the refrigerator for several hours or overnight. (When it is completely cool, you may cover it.)

15. After several hours remove the soup, and the lamb from the refrigerator. Using a slotted spoon, skim the top of the soup to remove the extra fat which will have hardened on the surface.

16. Heat the soup on the stove over medium high heat, stirring occasionally, until it is heated through.

17. To serve, place the desired portion of lamb into a bowl, top with heaping spoonfuls of the vegetables and ladle the hot broth over the top.

EGGPLANT STEW

This stew makes a lovely side dish, but you can easily turn it into a beautiful one pot meal. Just toss in some cooked shrimp, or some bite sized pieces of cooked chicken, lamb, beef, or pork, at step 12. It's an ideal way to turn yesterday's leftovers into something new and exciting for tonight's dinner.

Yield: 4-6 cups

Ingredients:

- » 2-3 small eggplants, cubed
- » 2 tbsp. extra virgin olive oil
- » 1 onion, diced
- » 3 carrots, sliced into rounds
- » Pinch of salt
- » ½ tsp. cumin
- » ¼ tsp. turmeric
- » 2-3 pinches of ground ginger
- » 14 oz. crushed tomatoes

DIRECTIONS:

1. Pre-heat your oven to 425°F.

2. Line a cookie sheet with aluminum foil, and spray with cooking oil.

3. Place the cubed eggplant on the cookie sheet, in an even layer.

4. Spray the eggplant with more cooking spray.

5. Roast the eggplant for about 20 minutes or until tender, stirring after 10 minutes.

6. Set the roasted eggplant on the side.

7. In a large pot, warm the oil over a medium heat. When the oil is hot, but not smoking, add in the onions and the carrots.

8. Sprinkle a pinch of salt over the cooking vegetables. Continue to sauté them until the onions are translucent and yellow.

9. Remove the pot from the heat. Add in the spices, and mix well.

10. Add in the roasted eggplant, and gently mix again.

11. Add in the tomatoes and return the pot to medium heat.

12. Add salt and pepper to taste.

13. Stirring, bring to a hard simmer. Cover and cook, stirring occasionally, for another five minutes.

14. Serve hot.

SUPER CHARGED CHILI – STAGE 3 ONLY

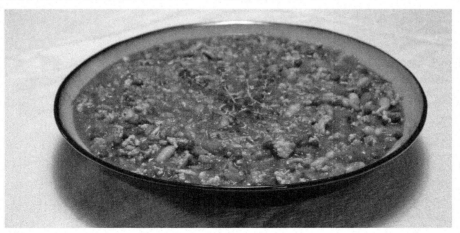

Ah, the enticing aroma of tomatoes and spices bubbling on the stove; the warming comfort in each rich forkful. Who doesn't love a good bowl of chili?

If you enjoy a great bowl of chili as much as I do, you have to try my special recipe. It's full of flavor, and I've amped up the nutritional value to make it super charged! It's brimming with proteins, fiber, antioxidants, healthy nutrients, and carefully selected spices known for their metabolism boosting, anti-inflammatory properties.

This recipe is on the mild side, so both young and old can dig in and enjoy! If you prefer a spicier dish, you can easily heat things up to your taste. Just increase the amount of chipotle and ancho chili powder in the recipe.

Yield: 10 cups

Serving size: 1 cup

Ingredients:

- » 1 1/2 lbs. ground meat, such as turkey, chicken, bison, or beef
- » 1 bell pepper, chopped
- » 2 tbsp. extra virgin olive oil
- » 1/2 clove of elephant garlic or 2 cloves garlic, minced
- » 1 large onion, chopped
- » 1 1/2 tbsp. paprika
- » 1/2 tbsp. dried oregano
- » 3/4 tsp turmeric powder
- » 1/8 tsp chipotle chili powder
- » 3/4 tsp cumin
- » 1/2 tsp ancho chili powder
- » 2 tsp dried cilantro
- » 2 tsp organic raw cacao powder
- » 1 cup filtered water

» 2 cans beans, 15 oz. each, rinsed and drained (I used cannellini and adzuki, because they were in my cupboard. You can use any 2 that you like.)

» 1 can diced tomatoes, 28 oz.

» 2 cups tomato puree

» salt & black pepper

DIRECTIONS:

1. Add the oil to a large, deep pan on the stove top.

2. Place the peppers in the pan. Stirring frequently, cook them over medium heat for 1-2 minutes, until they just slightly begin to soften.

3. Add the onions and garlic to the pan. Sprinkle with a pinch of salt. Continue to stir and cook until the onions become light yellow and translucent.

4. Shredding with your fingers, add the ground meat to the pan. Using your spoon to break the meat apart, continue cooking and stirring until the meat is cooked through.

5. Remove from the heat. Carefully drain all the liquid from your pan.

6. Sprinkle all the spices evenly over the mixture, and mix well.

7. Add the water to the pan, and mix well again.

8. Add the beans and tomato products to your pan.

9. Mix well, cover, and return to medium-high heat.

10. Allow mixture to come to a slow boil. Lower the heat, and allow the covered chili to simmer for at least 5 minutes.

11. Uncover the chili. Add salt and pepper to taste.

12. On low heat, continue to cook the chili for an additional 5 minutes or so, to thicken.

13. Serve immediately.

Any leftovers may be stored under refrigeration, in a covered container. This chili tastes even better the next day!

VEGETARIAN CHILI – STAGE 3 ONLY

Going vegetarian one or two nights a week is a good way to save some money, and to get some extra fiber into your meal.

This vegetarian chili is a big hit at my house, and is great served with my biscuit recipe. We like it mild at our house. If you want to spice things up a little, just increase the chili powder or add some seeded and chopped chilies, jalapenos, or poblanos to the bell peppers in recipe.

Yield: 11 cups

Serving size: 1 cup

Ingredients:

» 1 green bell pepper

» 1 red bell pepper

» 2 stalks of celery

» 3 large carrots, washed and peeled

» 5 small zucchinis

» 1 1/2 cups chopped mushrooms

» 1 large onion

» 4 cloves of garlic

» 15.5 oz. can adzuki beans, rinsed and drained

» 15.5 oz. can black beans, rinsed and drained

» 1 1/2 tbsp. paprika

» 3/4 tsp cumin

» 3/4 tsp ancho chili powder

» 2 tsp dried cilantro

- » 1/2 tsp dried oregano
- » 1/2 tsp turmeric powder
- » 1/4 cup filtered water
- » 28 oz. can crushed tomatoes
- » 3 tbsp. extra virgin olive oil
- » salt and pepper

DIRECTIONS:

1. Rinse, dry, and chop all the vegetables. Mince the garlic.
2. Place the oil and all the prepared vegetables, except for the beans, into a ceramic non-stick pan.
3. Season with salt and pepper to taste.
4. Cook over medium-low heat, stirring frequently, until the onions are translucent and the vegetables begin to cook and release their liquids.
5. Turn off the heat and sprinkle the spices evenly over the vegetables. Stir to evenly coat.
6. Add the water and beans. Mix well after each addition.
7. Add the tomatoes. Mix well, cover, and return to medium heat.
8. Allow the chili to simmer, covered, for about 5 minutes.
9. Uncover, lower the heat, and cook, stirring occasionally for another 5-10 minutes. This will allow the chili to thicken.

Enjoy with your favorite toppings and sides.

Store cooled chili in a covered container in the refrigerator for 3-4 days.

SAMBUSIK – STAGE 3 ONLY

Inspired by the same turnover recipe as the burger (recipe found in the entrée section), this version is more like a chili, or a sloppy joe. I often make it when I'm in a hurry to get a nice meal on the table, and the family loves it! You can serve it with a big salad and some biscuits (recipe found in the baking section), for a killer meal!

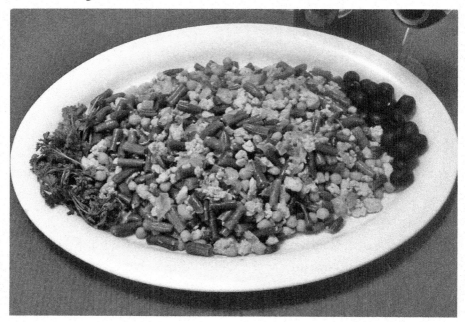

Yields: 4 servings

Ingredients:

- » 1 lb. fresh or frozen vegetables such as broccoli, cauliflower, or green beans, cooked al dente
- » 1 lb. ground turkey, chicken, beef, or bison
- » 1 large onion, diced
- » 2 tbsp. extra virgin olive oil
- » 15 oz. can of garbanzo beans, rinsed & drained
- » ½ cup water
- » 1/2 tsp cumin
- » 1/4 tsp turmeric
- » ½-1 tsp sea salt

» 1/8 tsp ground ginger

» 1/4 tsp black pepper

DIRECTIONS:

1. In a large sauté pan, heat the oil over medium heat until hot, but not smoking.

2. Add the onion to the pan and cook until the onion is translucent.

3. Shredding with your fingers, add the ground meat to the pan. Using your spoon to break the meat apart, continue cooking and stirring until the meat is cooked through.

4. Remove from the heat. Carefully drain all the liquid from your pan.

5. Sprinkle all the spices evenly over the mixture, and mix well.

6. Add the water to the pan, and mix well again.

7. Add the beans and the vegetables to the pan.

8. Mix well, cover, and return to medium heat.

9. Cook covered until heated through.

10. Uncover, and continue to cook for a few more minutes, stirring often. When most of the liquid has cooked down and the sambusik has thickened, it is done.

11. Serve immediately.

VEGETABLES AND SIDES

ROASTED ACORN SQUASH OR PIE PUMPKINS

These two winter gourds are brimming with vitamins, like vitamins C and A, and minerals like potassium and magnesium. They are a delicious way to get in your daily dose of orange colored foods.

Yield: Depends on the size and quantity of gourds used.

Serving size: ½ cup cooked

DIRECTIONS:

1. Pre-heat the oven to 425°F.
2. Line a baking sheet with aluminum foil.
3. Wash the outside of your squash/pumpkin with clean water.
4. With a sharp knife cut your squash or pumpkin in half. One half should have the stem, the other half would be the bottom.
5. With your hands, break off the long stem on the pumpkin. You should not have to bother with the stem on the acorn squash, unless it is overly long.
6. With a spoon, scoop out the seeds from the center. You may save them for toasting later, if you like.
7. Rub the interior cups with coconut oil or butter and place them cup side down on the prepared baking sheets.
8. Give the shells a thin coating of whichever fat you choose for the cups.
9. Place the baking sheet into the hot oven and bake for about 40-45 minutes or until the squash/pumpkin is easily pierced with a fork.
10. At this point, the pumpkin can be removed from the oven and served. If you are roasting acorn squash, you can either remove it from the oven and serve it, or you can turn the cups over, sprinkle them with some cinnamon, and bake for a few more minutes.

Both these vegetables are so versatile, you can serve them with cinnamon and butter, or with salt and pepper. The acorn squash cups make perfect containers for fillings like chili, or stews. Both go great with nuts, and nut butters, too.

BEET GREENS, BLANCHED & SAUTÉED

Beet greens are loaded with vitamins, including vitamins K, A, and C. They're also a great source of minerals such as magnesium, iron, and copper, but the benefits of eating beet greens don't stop there. They're also full of health promoting flavonoids, and phytonutrients. They're a good source of fiber, and they taste great! To save time, you can purchase fresh organic garlic that is already peeled for you.

Serves 4

Ingredients:

>> 8 bunches of beet greens

>> A large bowl of ice water

>> 6 cloves of garlic, peeled and chopped

>> 2-3 tbsps. extra virgin olive oil

>> salt and pepper

DIRECTIONS:

1. Wash your beet greens, and completely remove the center stem on each leaf.

2. Blanch the greens in boiling salted water, for about 2 minutes or until they are wilted.

3. Drain the greens and shock them in the bowl of ice water to stop the cooking process.

4. Drain the greens and squeeze out any excess water.

5. Heat the oil in a large sauté pan over a medium heat.

6. When the oil is hot, but not smoking, add the garlic to the pan.

7. Cook the garlic until it is fragrant.

8. Add the greens to the pan and cook until heated through.

9. Season with salt and pepper to taste.

10. Serve immediately.

CAULIFLOWER FRIED RICE

This recipe is a great way to make cauliflower that the whole family will love. You can serve it as a side dish, or you can toss in some leftover chicken, shrimp, beef, or pork, and turn this dish into a simple one pot dinner.

Serves: 4-5 people

Ingredients:

» 1 head of cauliflower, washed

» 1 tbsp. extra virgin olive oil

» 2 large organic pastured eggs

» ¾ cup frozen peas

» 2 small carrots, washed, peeled, and shredded

» 3 cloves of garlic, minced

» ¼ of a large onion, minced

» salt and pepper

» 2-3 tbsp. gluten free soy sauce/tamari sauce

Directions:

1. Cut the cauliflower into large wedges, which are small enough to fit through the feeding tube of a food processor.

2. Process the cauliflower pieces, one at a time, using the shredding blade of a food processor.

3. Heat the oil in a large sauté pan, over a medium heat.

4. Add all the vegetables except the garlic to the pan. Cook for 3-4

minutes, or until the cauliflower starts to get tender.

5. Add the garlic, and season to taste with salt and pepper. Cook until the garlic is fragrant, for about 30 seconds.

6. Push the vegetables to the sides of the pan. Cook and scramble the eggs in the cleared center part of the pan.

7. Toss the eggs into the vegetables, and drizzle the rice with the tamari sauce. Toss again to incorporate.

8. Serve hot.

SAUTÉED CABBAGE

This is a quick 5 ingredient dish that pairs nicely with pork, lamb, or beef. You can use white cabbage, purple cabbage, or shredded Brussel's sprouts to make this recipe.

Yield: 4-6 servings

Ingredients:

» 2 lbs. of shredded slaw mix, shredded red cabbage, or shredded Brussel's sprouts

» 2 tbsp. of extra virgin olive oil or butter

» 1 onion, sliced thinly

» 1 tbsp. caraway seeds

» Salt & pepper

» 1 tbsp. raw apple cider vinegar (optional)

DIRECTIONS:

1. Heat the oil in a large sauté pan over medium heat, for just a few seconds.

2. Add in the onions, the cabbage, and the seeds.

3. Cook, stirring constantly, until the cabbage wilts and is tender. If you are having issues with the cabbage not wilting, cover the pan

with a lid for a few moments. This will steam the vegetables and help them wilt.

4. Remove the pan from the heat, add in the vinegar, and toss well.

5. Season with salt and pepper to taste.

6. Toss again to be sure flavors are equally distributed, and serve.

EGGPLANT PARMESAN

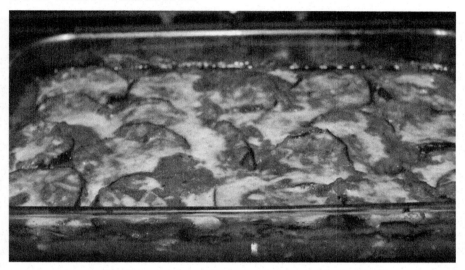

This recipe is delicious, with or without the cheese. Serve it with cheese on special occasions, and omit the cheese for every day fare. Turn it into a yummy dinner entrée by adding in layers of your favorite browned ground meat, such as beef, bison, or lamb. The leftovers are wonderful for lunch, too.

Yield: 8 servings

Ingredients:

» 3 medium eggplants

» 8 ounces of mozzarella cheese

» 2 jars of premium tomato basil style tomato sauce (with no added sugar or sweeteners) or 5 cups of homemade tomato sauce

» onion powder

» garlic powder

» dried oregano

» dried basil

DIRECTIONS:

1. Preheat your oven to 425°F.

2. Line 2 large baking trays with foil, and coat them lightly with cooking spray.

3. Slice the eggplant into about 1/8" rounds, and place them onto the greased baking sheets.

4. Spray them lightly with the cooking spray, and sprinkle them with the spices.

5. Bake the slices in the preheated oven for about 10 minutes. Flip them over and continue baking for another 10 minutes or until lightly browned and tender.

6. While they are baking, grate your mozzarella, and coat the bottom of your lasagna pan generously with sauce.

7. When the eggplant slices are done, take them out of the oven, and reduce the heat down to 350° F.

8. Layer the browned eggplant slices over the sauce in a single layer. Top with more sauce, and about a third of the cheese.

9. Continue layering in this way until you are out of eggplant.

10. Finish topping your eggplant parmesan with a last layer of sauce and cheese.

11. Spoon additional sauce around the edges of the pan, and over any exposed ends of eggplant.

12. Cover the lasagna pan with foil, and place in the center rack of your oven.

13. Bake covered for 45 minutes.

14. Uncover and bake for another 15 minutes.

15. When it is done, the sauce will be bubbly, and the cheese will be melted and light golden.

16. Allow the eggplant to cool for a few minutes before serving.

ROASTED SPAGHETTI SQUASH

Spaghetti squash is wonderful! It's low in carbs, and so versatile. It can be served with a nice marinara, alfredo, or pesto sauce. It's also good with butter, or olive oil and garlic. It's just as simple to make as roasted acorn squash. The most difficult part is cutting it open.

Yield: Depends on the size and quantity of gourds used.

Serving size: 1 cup cooked

DIRECTIONS:

1. Pre-heat the oven to 425°F.

2. Line a baking sheet with aluminum foil.

3. Wash the outside of your squash with clean water.

4. With a sharp knife, cut your squash in half, length wise, from stem to stern. You want to end up with two shallow ovals, not two cups. This part can be can be a little tricky. Use a sharp knife to pierce the squash in the center, and cut in one direction. Then, re-pierce the squash with the knife, and cut in the opposite direction. Flip the squash over, and repeat on the other side. If your knife gets stuck, carefully and gently tap the squash on the cutting board to release it.

5. With a spoon, scoop out the seeds from the center. You may save them for toasting later, if you like.

6. Rub the interior with coconut oil or butter, and place them flesh side down on the prepared baking sheets.

7. Give the shells a thin coating of coconut oil or butter.

8. Place the baking sheet into the hot oven and bake for about 40-45 minutes, or until the squash is easily pierced with a fork.

9. At this point, remove the squash from the oven. Let it cool just long enough so that you can safely handle it. Use a fork to scrape along the insides of the squash the long way. This will release the spaghetti-like strands.

10. Scoop the strands into a bowl or serving platter, and top with your choice of sauce.

11. Store any leftovers in the refrigerator, in a covered container.

SWEET POTATO LATKES – STAGE 3 ONLY

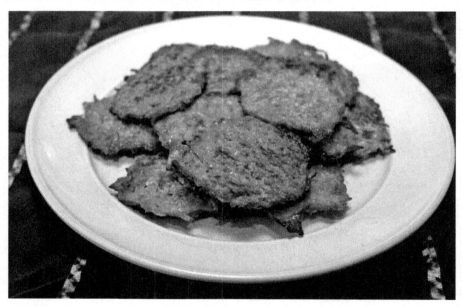

Yield: 30 latkes

Ingredients:

- » 2 lb. sweet potatoes
- » 6 large pastured eggs

» 3 tbsp. coconut flour

» 2 tsp. soda

» sea salt and black pepper

DIRECTIONS:

1. Preheat the oven to 350° F.

2. Line a baking sheet with foil or parchment paper. Grease the top of the liner.

3. Wash, peel, and grate the potatoes. (I use my food processor's grating blade for this step, but you can buy sweet potatoes already shredded, or you can grate them by hand if you like.)

4. Mix all the ingredients in a large bowl; add salt and pepper to taste.

5. With your hands, form the mixture into little pancakes, and place them one by one onto the baking sheet.

6. Spray them evenly with cooking spray.

7. Place the baking sheet onto the center rack of the hot oven.

8. Bake for 15 minutes. Using a metal spatula, flip the pancakes over and bake for another 12-15 minutes, until they are done. The finished pancakes should be golden brown on both sides.

ZUCCHINI NOODLES

This recipe is simple, and these "noodles" are another great replacement for pasta. You can serve them with tomato sauce, pesto, or just plain. For this recipe, you'll need a spiralizer, or you can purchase zucchini which has already been spiralized at most supermarkets.

Yield: 3-4 servings

Ingredients:

» 3 medium zucchinis, washed and spiralized

» 2-3 tbsp. extra virgin olive oil

» 3 cloves of garlic, peeled and minced

» Salt and pepper

DIRECTIONS:

1. In a large sauté pan, heat the oil over a medium heat for a few seconds.

2. Add the garlic and the zucchini to the pan.

3. Cook stirring gently, until the noodles are the desired tenderness. I keep mine a little on the al dente side so they don't become too mushy.

4. Add salt and pepper to taste, top with desired sauce or toppings.

ENTRÉES

ITALIAN FESTIVAL BURGERS WITH PEPPERS AND ONIONS

Inspired by the sweet Italian sausage & pepper sandwiches often found at summer festivals and street fairs, this recipe takes that classic flavor combination and gives it new appeal!

Yield: 4 burgers, approximately 4oz each when cooked

Ingredients:

- » 20 oz. package of ground turkey, chicken, beef, or bison
- » 1 tbsp. paprika
- » 1 tsp garlic powder
- » 1 tsp onion powder
- » 1 1/2 tsp fennel seeds
- » 1/2 tsp dried oregano
- » 1/2 tsp dried thyme
- » 1/2 tsp sea salt
- » 1/4 tsp black pepper
- » 1/4 tsp cumin

DIRECTIONS:

1. Place all the ingredients into a large bowl, mixing well to completely incorporate.
2. Form into four large patties.
3. Place patties on a plate, cover, and place in the refrigerator.
4. Prepare the pepper & onion topping as described in the recipe below.
5. When the topping is done, remove it from the heat, cover, and set aside.
6. Remove the burgers from the refrigerator, and grill over medium heat to desired doneness, or until a meat thermometer inserted

into the middle reaches over 165F.

7. Top with sautéed peppers & onions, and serve on artisan rolls. (recipe included in the baking section).

SAUTÉED PEPPERS & ONIONS

Ingredients:

» 2 medium red bell peppers, sliced into thin strips, about 1/4-½ inch wide.

» 1 medium green bell pepper, sliced into thin strips, about 1/4-½ inch wide.

» 1 large sweet yellow onion, julienned

» 2 tbsp. extra virgin olive oil

» 1/4 tsp dried basil

DIRECTIONS:

1. Heat oil in a sauté pan over medium heat, until hot but not smoking.

2. Add the peppers to the pan, and cook for a minute or two, stirring constantly.

3. Add in the onion and continue to cook, stirring constantly, until the peppers begin to soften, and the onions become translucent and start to yellow just a bit.

4. Mix well, and cover the pan for about a minute, stirring occasionally.

5. Sprinkle in the basil during the last few seconds of cooking.

6. The mixture is cooked when the peppers are soft, and the onions are a deep golden yellow. Be careful not to burn your onions, as they cook quickly toward the end.

7. Store cooled leftovers in a covered container, in the refrigerator.

TACO BURGERS

These tasty burgers have a fun southwestern flair that the whole family will love. Make them and turn your next family barbeque into a fiesta!

Yield: 4 burgers, approximately 4oz each when cooked

Ingredients:

- » 20 oz. package of ground turkey, chicken, beef, or bison
- » 1/8 cup shallots, finely minced
- » 2 tsp paprika
- » 1 tsp onion powder
- » 1 tsp garlic powder
- » 1 tsp dried oregano
- » 1 tsp dried cilantro
- » 1/2 tsp cumin
- » 1/4 tsp turmeric
- » 1/4 tsp ancho chili powder
- » 1/8 tsp chipotle chili powder
- » 1/2 tsp sea salt
- » 1/8 tsp black pepper

DIRECTIONS:

1. Place all the ingredients into a large bowl, mixing well to completely incorporate.
2. Form into four large patties.
3. Grill over medium heat to desired doneness, or until a meat thermometer inserted into the middle reaches over 165F.
4. Serve wrapped in lettuce or inside of tortillas, or artisan rolls (both recipes included in the baking section). Top with salsa or taco sauce, and your favorite sandwich toppings such as, avocado, sliced tomatoes, olives, and lettuce.

GYRO BURGERS

What can I say, who doesn't love a gyro sandwich?

Yield: 4 burgers, approximately 4oz each when cooked

Ingredients:

- » 10 oz. package of ground lamb
- » 10 oz. package of ground beef, or bison
- » 1/4 cup finely minced onion
- » 1/2 tsp allspice
- » 1/2 tsp coriander
- » 1/2 tsp cumin
- » 1/2 tsp sea salt
- » 1/8 tsp black pepper

DIRECTIONS:

1. Place all the ingredients into a large bowl, mixing well to completely incorporate.
2. Form into four large patties.
3. Place patties on a plate, cover, and place in the refrigerator.
4. Prepare the tzatziki sauce recipe, as described below.
5. When the tzatziki sauce is done, place it in a covered container, and refrigerate.
6. Remove the burgers from the refrigerator, and grill over medium heat to desired doneness, or until a meat thermometer inserted into the middle reaches over 165F.
7. Serve wrapped in lettuce, or inside of tortillas or artisan rolls (recipes included in the baking section). Top with tzatziki sauce, and add your favorite sandwich toppings, such as sliced tomatoes, red onions, and lettuce.

TZATZIKI SAUCE

Yield: 4 servings

Ingredients:

- » 8 oz. plain full-fat, grass fed Greek yogurt
- » 1 cucumber, seeded and chopped
- » 1 tbsp. red wine vinegar
- » 1 tbsp. fresh dill
- » 1/2 tsp garlic powder
- » sea salt and black pepper to taste

DIRECTIONS:

1. Place all the ingredients into a food processor that has been fitted with a steel blade.
2. Process for 3-4 minutes, or until the sauce is fairly smooth and has thinned down a little.
3. Store in a covered container in the refrigerator.

SAMBUSIK BURGERS

This burger recipe was inspired by the exotic flavors of the Middle East and the Mediterranean. The flavor profile is typical of a meat turnover often enjoyed in these parts of the world, called sambusik. I have paired this burger with my own twist on a traditional yogurt dipping sauce, which is also served in these areas.

Yield: 4 burgers, approximately 4oz each when cooked

Ingredients:

- » 20 oz. package of ground turkey, chicken, beef, or bison
- » 1/3 cup onion, finely minced
- » 1/2 tsp cumin
- » 1/4 tsp turmeric

» 1/4 tsp sea salt

» 1/8 tsp ground ginger

» 1/8 tsp black pepper

DIRECTIONS:

1. Place all the ingredients into a large bowl, mixing well to completely incorporate.

2. Form into four large patties.

3. Place patties on a plate, cover, and place in the refrigerator.

4. Prepare the yogurt dipping sauce, as described below.

5. When the dipping sauce is done, place it in a covered container, and refrigerate.

6. Remove the burgers from the refrigerator, and grill over medium heat to desired doneness, or until a meat thermometer inserted into the middle reaches over 165F.

7. Serve wrapped in lettuce or inside of tortillas, or artisan rolls (recipes included in the baking section). Top with yogurt sauce and lettuce.

MINTY LEMON YOGURT DIPPING SAUCE

Yield: 8 servings

Ingredients:

» 8 oz. plain full-fat, grass fed Greek yogurt

» 1 tbsp. fresh mint leaves, chopped

» 1/4 tsp ground coriander

» juice from 1/2 of a fresh lemon

» 2 1/2 tbsp. extra virgin olive oil

» sea salt and black pepper to taste

DIRECTIONS:

1. Place all the ingredients into a food processor that has been fitted with a steel blade.

2. Process for 3-4 minutes, scraping down the bowl as needed, until the sauce is smooth and shiny, like mayonnaise.

3. Store in a covered container in the refrigerator

KEFTA MEATLOAF – STAGE 3 ONLY

This meatloaf recipe was inspired by keftedes, which are small spiced Greek meatballs. The recipe adds some pizzazz, elevating meatloaf up to new levels of enjoyment.

Yield: 4-6 servings

Ingredients:

- » 1 lb. ground beef
- » 1 lb. ground lamb
- » 2 large eggs
- » ¼ cup filtered water
- » 1/3 a medium onion, minced
- » 5 cloves of garlic, peeled and minced
- » 1 tbsp. dried dill
- » 1 tsp. dried oregano
- » ½ tsp. cumin
- » 1 tbsp. fresh lemon juice
- » ¾ tsp. sea salt
- » ½ tsp. black pepper
- » ¼ cup garbanzo bean flour
- » 1 – 28 oz. can, diced tomatoes
- » ½ cup good red wine

DIRECTIONS:

1. Pre-heat the oven to 350°F

2. In a large bowl, combine all the ingredients, except for the tomatoes and the wine.

3. With your hands, form the meat into a loaf, and carefully place into a glass lasagna dish. You can perfect the shape of your loaf once it's in the dish.

4. Add some water to the bottom of the dish. It should be about ¼-½" deep.

5. Pour the diced tomatoes over the top of the meat loaf.

6. Cover the dish tightly with aluminum foil, and bake on the center rack of the pre-heated oven for 1 hour.

7. After an hour, remove the meat loaf from the oven and pour the wine over the top.

8. Return to the oven uncovered, and cook for another 45 minutes, until done. The center should read 170F or higher, on a cooking thermometer.

ITALIAN STYLE MEATBALLS IN RUSTIC TOMATO SAUCE – STAGE 3 ONLY

Yield: 18 Meatballs

Servings: 4-6

Added sugar per serving: trace amount

The fragrant smell of tomatoes, onions, and peppers cooking always takes me back to my grandmother René's kitchen. Her home was a place full of love, and it always smelled like good things cooking. For me and my family, this recipe represents some real comfort food any time of the year. It's pretty simple to whip up, it's hearty, and good for your body & soul. I hope your family enjoys it as much as mine does.

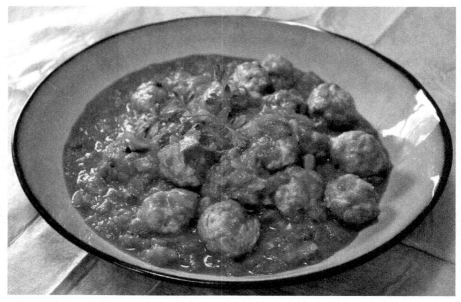

Ingredients:

» 32oz. ground turkey, chicken, beef, or bison

» 1 Tbsp. paprika

» 1 tsp. garlic powder

» 1 tsp. onion powder

» 1 1/4 tsp. fennel seeds

» 3/4 tsp. dried oregano

» 1/2 tsp. dried thyme

» 1/2 tsp. sea salt

» 1/4 tsp. black pepper

» 1/4 tsp. cumin

» 1/3-1/2 cup garbanzo bean flour or almond meal

» 2 large egg

» 1/2 cup - 1 cup water

» 2 Tbsp. extra virgin olive oil

» 1 red bell pepper, chopped

» 1 large sweet onion, chopped

» 28 oz. can crushed tomatoes, no salt added

» 12 basil leaves, roughly torn

» 1 tbsp. fresh oregano

» 1/2 tbsp. fresh parsley leaves

» 1 tsp. honey

» 1 tsp. aged balsamic vinegar

» Additional sea salt & black pepper to taste

DIRECTIONS:

1. In a large bowl, combine the first twelve ingredients and 2 tbsp. of the water. Mix well to completely combine.

2. Using wet hands, form the mixture into 18 small meatballs of equal size. Place each meatball on a large plate and set aside. If the mixture is too loose to form meatballs, add in a bit more garbanzo bean flour or almond meal.

3. Pour the olive oil into a large, sauté pan.

4. Place the pan on the stove top, over a medium heat, and add in the peppers.

5. Cook the peppers for a minute or two, then add in the onions, garlic, and a pinch of sea salt.

6. Stir constantly until the onions become translucent but are not browned.

7. Pour in the tomatoes.

8. Slowly stir in a 1/2 cup or so of the water, a little at a time, until the sauce reaches the desired consistency.

9. When the sauce begins to bubble, carefully add in the meatballs, one at a time.

10. Place the lid on the pan. Lower the heat slightly, and allow the

meatballs to cook at a boil for five minutes. Gently stir the meatballs occasionally, to ensure that the sauce covers the meatballs and they are not sticking to the pan.

11. After five minutes, reduce the heat to a simmer, then stir in the honey and the vinegar.

12. Cook covered for about 20-25 minutes, until the meat is cooked through and tender.

13. Towards the last few minutes of cooking, add in the fresh herbs and additional salt & pepper to taste.

14. Store any leftovers in a covered container in the refrigerator, after they have cooled a bit.

ALMOST HOMEMADE ITALIAN STYLE MEATBALLS IN MARINARA SAUCE

This recipe is perfect for those days when you want to get a nice dinner on the table, without too much fussing. Serve them over zucchini noodles or cooked spaghetti squash. You can also find pasta made with only black beans or lentils at the grocery store.

Yield: 18 Meatballs

Servings: 4-6

Ingredients:

» 32oz. ground turkey, chicken, beef, or bison

» 1 tbsp. paprika

» 1 tsp. garlic powder

» 1 tsp. onion powder

» 1 1/4 tsp. fennel seeds

» 3/4 tsp. dried oregano

» 1/2 tsp. dried thyme

» 1/2 tsp. sea salt

» 1/4 tsp. black pepper

» 1/4 tsp. cumin

» 1/3-1/2 cup garbanzo bean flour or almond meal

» 2 large egg

» 2 tbsp. filtered water

» 40 oz. Organic jarred Marinara sauce, (with no added sugar)

DIRECTIONS:

1. Place all the ingredients, except the sauce, into a large bowl. Mix well to completely combine.

2. Using wet hands, form the mixture into 18 small meatballs of equal size. Place each meatball on a large plate and set aside. If the mixture is too loose to form meatballs, add in a bit more garbanzo bean flour or almond meal.

3. Pour the sauce into a large sauté pan. Place the pan on the stove top over a medium heat.

4. When the sauce begins to bubble, carefully add in the meatballs, one at a time.

5. Place the lid on the pan. Lower the heat slightly, and allow the meatballs to cook at a boil for five minutes. Gently stir the meatballs occasionally, to ensure that the sauce covers the meatballs, and they are not sticking to the pan.

6. After five minutes, reduce the heat to a simmer.

7. Cook covered for about 20-25 minutes, until the meat is cooked through and tender.

8. Store any leftovers in a covered container in the refrigerator, after they have cooled a bit.

STUFFED ACORN SQUASH – STAGE 3 ONLY

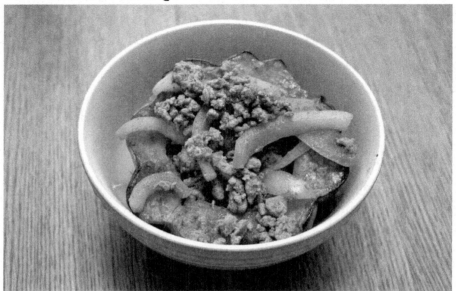

The sweetness of the acorn squash goes very well with this savory sausage filling. This hearty dish really hits the spot after a busy day.

Yield: 4 servings

- » 20 oz. ground turkey, chicken, beef, or bison
- » 1 large bell pepper; washed, seeded, and sliced
- » ½ a Vidalia onion, peeled and thinly sliced
- » 2 tbsp. extra virgin olive oil
- » 1 tbsp. paprika
- » 1 tsp garlic powder
- » 1 tsp onion powder
- » 1 1/2 tsp fennel seeds
- » 1/2 tsp dried oregano
- » 1/2 tsp dried thyme
- » 1/2 tsp sea salt

» 1/4 tsp black pepper

» 1/4 tsp cumin

» 2 whole acorn squashes

» 1/3 cup filtered water

DIRECTIONS:

1. Prepare the squashes and roast them as per the Roasted Acorn Squash or Pie Pumpkins recipe. While the squash is roasting, prepare the filling.

To prepare the filling:

1. Place the oil into a large sauté pan, over medium heat. Heat the oil until it's hot but not smoking.

2. When the oil is hot, place the peppers in the pan. Stirring frequently, cook them over medium heat for 1-2 minutes, until they just slightly begin to soften.

3. Add the onions to the pan. Continue to stir, and cook until the onions become light yellow and translucent.

4. Shredding with your fingers, add the ground meat to the pan. Using your spoon to break the meat apart, continue cooking and stirring until the meat is cooked through.

5. Remove from the heat. Carefully drain all the liquid from your pan.

6. Sprinkle all the spices evenly over the mixture, and mix well.

7. Add the water to the pan, and mix well again.

8. Cook for a few minutes, stirring often, until the spices are well combined and the liquid has mostly cooked out.

9. When the acorn squash is done, fill each squash half with some of the filling, and serve immediately.

Easy Meat Sauce

For those nights when comfort food is called for, and time is of the essence. This meal should take less than 20 minutes to prepare. Serve over leftover vegetables, zucchini noodles, cooked spaghetti squash, or store-bought lentil pasta. To complete the meal, serve it with a large green salad on the side.

Yield: 3-4 servings

Ingredients:

» 16 oz. ground turkey, chicken, beef, bison, or lamb

» 24 oz. organic jarred marinara sauce, (with no added sugar)

» 2 tbsp. extra virgin olive oil

» Optional: chopped onions, chopped bell peppers, sliced mushrooms, ½ cup cooked peas & carrots.

DIRECTIONS:

1. Place the oil into a large sauté pan, over medium heat.

2. Heat the oil until it's hot but not smoking.

3. When the oil is hot, add in the optional onions, mushrooms, or peppers. You can use them individually, or in any combination. Cook them for a minute or two, until they begin to soften. Next, add the ground meat to the pan. If you are not using any raw vegetables, place the ground meat directly into the oil.

4. Cook the meat, stirring constantly, and breaking the clumps apart with a large spoon or spatula, until it is brown and almost cooked through.

5. Remove from the heat, and carefully drain the excess oils from the pan.

6. Pour the sauce into the pan, and return to a medium heat.

7. Cook covered for 5 minutes. The sauce should be gently bubbling during these 5 minutes, adjust your heat up or down, if necessary.

8. After 5 minutes, remove the cover and lower the heat all the way down. Now you can add in the cooked peas & carrots, if you like. Allow the meat sauce to cook at a simmer stirring occasionally, for about 5 minutes or until it reaches the desired thickness and the peas & carrots are heated through.

CHICKEN FAJITAS

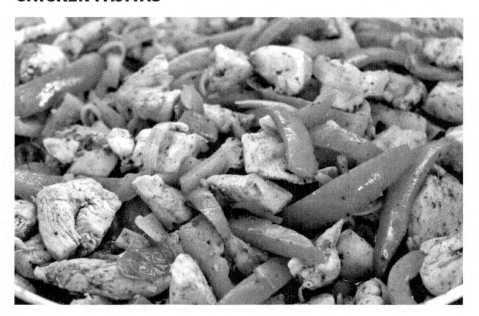

Make tonight's meal a Mexican fiesta! Serve these wonderful fajitas with fresh tortillas and homemade guacamole; you'll find the recipes in the baking and dip sections of this book. Round out the meal with some salsa, and a big green salad. Olé!

Yield: 4-6 servings

Ingredients:

- » 3 boneless and skinless chicken breasts, cut into bite sized strips
- » 3 red bell peppers, cut into strips
- » 2 onions, thinly sliced
- » 5 oz. baby portabella mushrooms, thinly sliced

» 1 cup grape tomatoes, halved

» 4 tbsp. extra virgin olive oil, divided

» 1 ½ tbsp. paprika

» 2 tsp. dried cilantro

» ¾ tsp cumin

» ¾ tsp. ancho chili powder

» ¼ tsp. garlic powder

» ¼ tsp. dried oregano

» ¼ cup filtered water

» sea salt and black pepper to taste

DIRECTIONS:

1. Place 2 tbsps. of the oil into a large sauté pan, over medium heat. Heat the oil until it's hot but not smoking.

2. When the oil is hot, add the peppers to the pan. Cook the peppers for a minute or two, stirring often. Next, add the mushrooms and onions to the pan.

3. Continue to cook the vegetables until the onions are translucent and the mushrooms begin to release their liquid.

4. Remove from the heat. Using a slotted spoon, spoon the vegetables into a large bowl.

5. Place the remaining 2 tbsps. of oil into the pan, and return to a medium heat. Heat the oil until it's hot but not smoking.

6. Carefully, add the chicken strips to the hot oil. Cook, stirring often, until the chicken is almost cooked through.

7. Cover the pan and continue to cook, stirring occasionally, until the chicken is tender and cooked through.

8. Toss the vegetables with the chicken in the pan. Sprinkle all the herbs and spices, except for the salt and pepper, over the top. Mix well.

9. Add the water to the pan. Mix well.

10. Cook uncovered for another minute or two, mixing occasionally, until the liquid is mostly cooked out. Season with salt and pepper to taste.

11. Serve immediately.

Hint: Use already cooked chicken, shrimp, or beef strips, for a super quick Mexican inspired meal.

CHICKEN CACCIATORE

My take on a classic Italian meal that you won't have to go to a restaurant to enjoy.

Yield: 4-6 servings

Ingredients:

» 4 boneless and skinless chicken breasts

» 2 tbsp. extra virgin olive oil

» 1 red bell pepper, thinly sliced into 1" strips

» 1 green bell pepper, thinly sliced into 1" strips

» ½ a Vidalia onion, thinly sliced

» 10 oz. of mushrooms, sliced

» 4 cloves of garlic, peeled and minced

» 1 can (28oz.) organic peeled whole tomatoes

» ½ tsp dried oregano

» ¾ tsp. dried basil

» ½ cup red wine

» ¾ cup medium black peppers

» Salt and black pepper

» optional: red pepper flakes, 3 oz. shredded mozzarella

DIRECTIONS:

1. Pre-heat the oven to 350°F.

2. In a medium sized bowl, squash the tomatoes up with your fingers, and set on the side.

3. Place the oil into a large sauté pan, over medium heat. Heat the oil until it's hot but not smoking.

4. When the oil is hot, add the onions, peppers, mushrooms, and garlic to the pan.

5. Cook until the onions are translucent.

6. Add the tomatoes, spices, olives, and the wine in with the cooking vegetables. Season to taste with salt, pepper, and red pepper flakes.

7. Cover the pan, and simmer for 1-2 minutes.

8. Ladle some of the sauce onto the bottom of a large, glass lasagna dish. Use enough sauce to cover the bottom of the dish, and arrange the chicken breasts on top of the sauce.

9. Carefully pour the rest of the sauce over the chicken.

10. Cover the dish tightly with aluminum foil.

11. Place the dish on the center rack of the pre-heated oven, and bake for 40 minutes.

12. After 40 minutes, uncover the chicken and bake for an additional 30 minutes, or until the chicken is fully cooked.

13. When the chicken is fully cooked you can serve it, or you can top it with the optional mozzarella, and place it under the broiler, until the cheese is melted and bubbly.

Hint: Leftover sauce and veggies are fantastic over your eggs at breakfast.

SPEEDY CASHEW CHICKEN

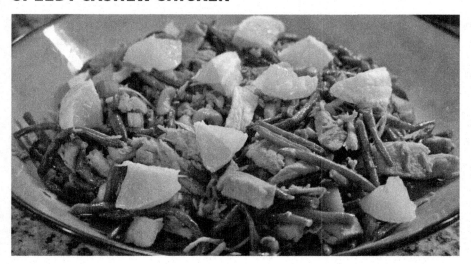

Craving Chinese tonight? This recipe is an unexpected way to repurpose leftover chicken or turkey.

Yield: 4 servings

Ingredients:

- » 2-10 oz. bags of frozen whole green beans
- » 8-10 cloves of garlic, peeled and minced
- » 6 stalks of celery, cleaned and chopped
- » 2 tbsp. coconut oil
- » 13 oz. cooked chicken or turkey
- » 2 ¼ tbsps. tamari sauce (gluten free soy sauce)
- » 3 tbsp. whole cashews
- » ½ cup filtered water
- » 1 orange, peeled, segmented, and cut into bite sized wedges
- » optional: red pepper flakes
- » optional: 4 tsp. organic raw honey – stage 3 only (Added sugar per serving: 1 tsp.)

DIRECTIONS:

1. In a large sauté pan over medium heat, cook the green beans, garlic, and celery until the beans are heated through, and the garlic is fragrant.

2. Toss in the chicken, the tamari, the water, and the orange segments (save about 10 pieces for the garnish), and the honey if you're using it.

3. Cook over medium heat until the vegetables and chicken are tender and heated through.

4. Toss in the cashews, and some red pepper flakes to taste.

5. Place into a large serving dish or into individual bowls, and garnish with the remaining orange pieces.

6. Serve immediately.

LEMONY MEDITERRANEAN CHICKEN

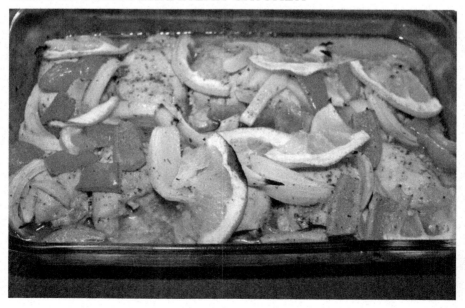

I love fresh lemons. I like them so much, I have been known to eat them like an orange right of the peel (they're especially good with a little salt), and in my house, people will complain if there isn't an ample amount of garlic incorporated into most of my dinner recipes. In this simple to make Mediterranean style chicken dish, I think you'll enjoy the way the flavors of the lemon slices, garlic, olive oil, and spices all blend together, and if you like lemon and garlic the way I do, then this is the chicken dish for you!

Yield: 5 Servings

Serving size: 2 thighs

Ingredients:

- » 10 organic, boneless, skinless chicken thighs
- » 1/4 cup extra virgin olive oil
- » 2 Tbsp. fresh lemon juice
- » 1 tsp. garlic powder
- » 1 Tbsp. dried oregano
- » 1/2 tsp. turmeric
- » 3/4 tsp. sea salt
- » 1/2 tsp. black pepper
- » 1 bell pepper, cut into 1" strips
- » 1/2 a large sweet onion, cut into 1" wedges
- » 1 fresh lemon, thinly sliced

DIRECTIONS:

1. Preheat the oven to 400°F.
2. In a bowl, combine the oil, lemon juice, and spices.
3. Spray the bottom of a 9 x 13 baking dish with cooking spray. Arrange the thighs in the dish, and brush them with the lemon juice mixture.
4. Place the peppers, onions, and lemon slices into the bowl with the remaining juice mixture, and toss well to coat.

5. Arrange the vegetables and lemon slices on top of the chicken, and pour the juice over the top.

6. Bake in the center rack of your oven for 30 minutes. Baste the chicken and vegetables with the pan drippings, and continue to cook for about another 10 minutes, until the chicken is cooked through. The thighs should reach above 165 F on a meat thermometer, and the juices should run clear.

ITALIAN STYLE CHICKEN CUTLETS

These are great on their own, or smothered in tomato sauce. Big kids, and little ones, will like the combination of crispy breading and tender chicken.

Yield: 8 chicken cutlets

Ingredients:

- » 4 boneless skinless split chicken breasts, or 8 thin sliced chicken cutlets
- » 2 cups of almond meal
- » 2 tbsp. flax meal
- » 1 tsp. onion powder
- » 1 ¼ tsp. garlic powder
- » 2 tsp. dried oregano
- » 1 ½ tsp. dried parsley
- » ½ tsp. dried basil
- » ½ tsp. paprika
- » ½ tsp. sea salt, or to taste
- » ¼ tsp. black pepper, or to taste
- » 2 large pastured eggs

DIRECTIONS:

1. Preheat the oven to 350°F.

2. Line a baking sheet with aluminum foil. Coat the baking sheet evenly with cooking spray.

3. With a sharp knife, carefully cut each chicken breast in half to create two thin cutlets. (Skip this step if you purchased already trimmed, thin chicken cutlets.)

4. In a small bowl, whisk the eggs.

5. In a shallow dish, combine the almond meal, the flax meal, and the spices. Mix well.

6. One by one, dip the chicken cutlets into the egg, and then into the almond meal breading.

7. Coat each cutlet evenly with breading on both sides, and place it onto the prepared baking sheet.

8. When all the cutlets are breaded and on the baking sheet, lightly coat them with cooking spray.

9. Place the baking sheet onto the center rack of the preheated oven, and bake for about 45 minutes, until done. Turn the cutlets over about half way through the cooking time, for crispier cutlets.

COCONUT SHRIMP

Yield: 4 Servings

Ingredients:

» 1 lb. large shrimp, tail on, peeled & cleaned

» 2 large pastured eggs, beaten

» 1 cup unsweetened shredded coconut

» 1/4 tsp garlic powder

» 1/4 tsp paprika

» 3/4 cup almond meal flour

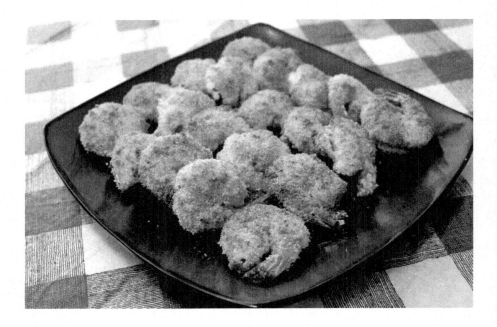

DIRECTIONS:

1. Preheat the oven to 425°F.

2. Line a baking sheet with foil, and spray evenly with cooking spray, to coat.

3. Place the coconut and spices into a large, shallow, rimmed dish, and mix with a fork until well combined.

4. Place the almond meal into a small bowl.

5. Place the eggs into another small bowl.

6. To bread the shrimp, dip one shrimp at a time into the almond meal, then into the egg. Gently shake off any extra egg, and then dip the shrimp into the coconut mixture.

7. Place each shrimp onto the baking sheet after they have been coated in breading, and spray lightly with cooking spray to coat.

8. Place on the center rack of the preheated oven, and bake for approx. 25-30 minutes, or until they are a deep golden brown and tender.

OVEN FRIED FISH

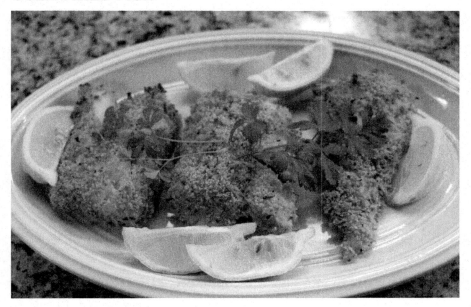

The kids will love this fish served with some HBC ketchup (recipe in condiment section of this book) on the side to dunk their fish into. You can also make a quick tartar sauce for the adults. Just add a squeeze of lemon juice, some chopped pickles, a little dill, and garlic powder to the HBC mayo recipe (also found in the condiment section) for a yummy, fresh tasting tartar sauce.

Yield: 4 servings

Ingredients:

- » 1 lb. wild white fish fillets, such as haddock, flounder, sole, or cod
- » 1 ½ cups hazelnut meal or almond meal
- » 1 tsp. garlic powder
- » 1 tsp. dried parsley
- » ¾ tsp. onion powder
- » 2 tsp. dried chives

» 2 tsp. paprika

» 1 large pastured egg

» sea salt & black pepper to taste

» coconut oil, or olive oil cooking spray

DIRECTIONS:

1. Pre-heat the oven to 425°F.

2. Line a baking sheet with aluminum foil, and coat evenly with cooking spray.

3. Place the egg into a bowl, and beat well with a fork.

4. Place the spices and nut meal into a shallow dish, or pan. Mix well to combine.

5. Cut your fish into smaller pieces, if necessary. Dip each piece one at a time, first into the egg and then into the seasoned nut meal. Be sure that both sides of the fish are evenly coated.

6. Place the fish on the baking sheet.

7. When all the fish is on the baking sheet, coat the pieces evenly with cooking spray.

8. Place the baking pan on the center rack of the pre-heated oven, and bake for 10-20 minutes depending on the thickness of the fish.

9. Remove the fish from the oven. With a spatula, gently flip each piece onto its other side. Return to the oven for 5-10 minutes to allow the coating to crisp.

10. Remove from the oven, and serve immediately.

SALMON WITH ROASTED BRUSSELS SPROUTS

This is a nice dish to serve to guests. The preparation is a snap, and cooking time is only around 30 minutes! If you'd like to, you can substitute the Brussels sprouts out for another green vegetable such as sautéed asparagus or steamed spinach.

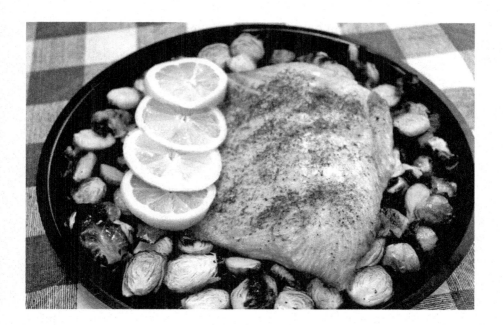

Yield: 4-6 servings

Ingredients:

» 1 1/2 lbs. fresh, wild salmon fillet

» 1/4 tsp garlic powder

» 1/4 tsp onion powder

» 1/4 tsp dried dill

» 1 lb. Brussels sprouts (washed, ends trimmed off, and cut in half vertically)

» 2 Tbsp. extra virgin olive oil

» 1 large wedge of fresh lemon

» salt and pepper

DIRECTIONS:

1. Preheat oven to 425°F.

2. Line two baking sheets with aluminum foil, and coat lightly with cooking spray.

3. Place salmon on one of the baking sheets, skin side down.

4. Evenly sprinkle the onion powder, garlic powder, and dill over the top of the fish.

5. Season with salt and pepper to taste.

6. Cover baking sheet with aluminum foil, completely enclosing the salmon.

7. Place the baking sheet on the center rack of the oven, leaving room for the Brussels sprouts.

8. In a large bowl, toss the Brussels sprouts with the olive oil.

9. Spread them onto the remaining baking sheet in a single layer.

10. Season with salt and pepper to taste, and place in the oven next to the salmon.

11. Cook salmon covered, for approx. 25-30 minutes or until almost cooked. Uncover, and continue to cook for 5 minutes, or until it is lightly browned on top. Salmon is completely cooked when the center is opaque, the fish flakes easily with a fork, and the internal temperature reaches above 145 degrees F.

12. When the Brussels sprouts are crispy, tender, and golden brown, remove them from the oven. The Brussels sprouts and the salmon should both be done around the same time.

13. Squeeze some fresh lemon juice over the salmon and the Brussels sprouts, and serve immediately. Garnish with fresh lemon wedges or slices if you like.

Hint: During the hot days of summer, you can serve the fish chilled, with fresh cucumber & tomato salad on the side.

ONION AND SAGE PORK ROAST

This is simplicity at its best, and you really can't mess it up. Just pour the liquid over the top, sprinkle with seasonings, set it, and forget it!

I love the flavor combo of onion and sage, but you could use just about any savory flavor combo that you like for example, garlic and rosemary; or garlic, onion, and oregano. You could even spread a thin layer of mustard over the top before adding your favorite seasonings. Have fun with it, and know tonight's dinner is going to be great!

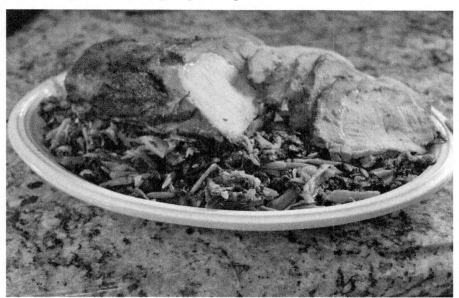

Yield: 6 servings

Serving Size: 4 ounces

Ingredients:

- » 3 lbs. boneless center cut pork loin
- » 7 oz. light beer, or 3oz. apple cider vinegar & 4oz. filtered water, or 7 oz. filtered water
- » turmeric powder
- » onion powder
- » dried sage
- » sea salt
- » black pepper

» extra virgin olive oil

DIRECTIONS:

1. Preheat oven the to 350°F.
2. Place the pork loin, fat side up, in the center of your roasting pan.
3. Pour the beer, cider mixture, or water over the roast.
4. Generously coat the roast with onion powder.
5. Sprinkle 2 pinches of turmeric over the roast.
6. Sprinkle generously with sage.
7. Season with salt and pepper.
8. Lightly drizzle with olive oil.
9. Place the roast into the preheated oven. Allow to cook for approximately 2 1/2 hours.

The roast is cooked when a thermometer placed near the center, reads above 165 F, the meat is tender, and the juices run clear. Serve with your favorite vegetables, and a nice salad. In the picture above, this roast is served over sautéed broccoli rabe with garlic.

CONDIMENTS, DIPS, & SPREADS

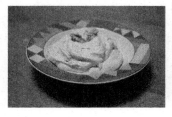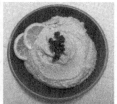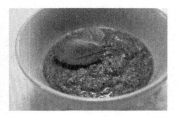

THANKSGIVING CRANBERRY SAUCE – STAGE 3 ONLY

For most people, thanksgiving just wouldn't be thanksgiving, without the cranberry sauce.

Yield: 3 ¼ cups

Serving size: 1 Tbsp.

Added sugar per serving: 1 tsp.

Ingredients:

» 12 oz. fresh cranberries, rinsed and picked through

» ½ cup fresh raspberries

» ½ cup fresh blackberries

» 2 large tangerines or 2 small oranges, peeled and seeded

» ½ cup filtered water

» 1 cup organic raw honey

DIRECTIONS:

1. Blend the tangerines and the water in a high-speed blender until smooth.

2. Place the blended tangerines and the remaining ingredients into a sauce pan.

3. Cook over a medium heat, stirring constantly for 18-20 minutes, or until the berries pop and the sauce thickens.

4. Chill for several hours or overnight. The sauce will continue to thicken and gel as it chills.

HBC KETCHUP – STAGE 3 ONLY

If ketchup is a major staple in your house, this is the recipe for you. It's amazingly simple to make, and the best part is you'll know exactly how much sugar is added. Which, by the way is very little, but you won't miss it one bit. This ketchup is as good, if not better, than any of the sugar filled, name brands.

Yield: 3 ¼ cups

Serving size: 2 tbsp.

Added sugar per serving: 1/6 tsp.

Ingredients:

- » 3-6 oz. cans of organic tomato paste
- » ½ cup organic raw apple cider vinegar
- » 1 tsp. garlic powder
- » 1 tbsp. organic raw honey
- » 2 tsp. sea salt
- » 1 pinch mustard powder
- » ½ tsp. hot sauce
- » 2 dashes ground cinnamon
- » 1 pinch allspice
- » 3 dashes paprika
- » ¾ cup filtered water

DIRECTIONS:

1. Place all the ingredients into a food processor that has been fitted with a steel blade, and process until smooth.
2. Scoop the ketchup into a glass container with a lid.
3. For the best flavor, chill overnight in the refrigerator. When it's first made, it tends to taste a little spicy, but it mellows out to a nice ketchup flavor overnight.
4. Store in a closed container in the refrigerator, as this ketchup contains no preservatives.

HBC MAYO

The only way I could find a mayonnaise that was sugar free, and made with pure extra virgin olive oil, was to create my own. Making your own mayonnaise might sound daunting, but it's really not very difficult. If you follow the directions carefully, you'll have the most delicious mayonnaise you've ever had, and it will only take a few minutes to make.

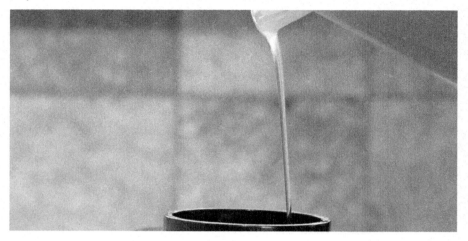

Yield: 2 cups

Ingredients:

- » 2 large pastured egg yolks
- » 1 ½ tbsp. organic raw apple cider vinegar
- » ½ tsp. salt
- » 1/8 tsp. dry mustard powder
- » 1-2/3 cup extra virgin olive oil

DIRECTIONS:

1. Place the egg yolks into the bowl of a food processor which has been fitted with a steel blade.

2. Process on the fastest setting for 1 minute. On my machine, it is the puree/mix button.

3. Pour the vinegar through the feed tube, and continue to process for 30 seconds more.

4. With the machine still running, pour the salt and mustard pow-

der into the feed tube. Then slowly begin to pour the olive oil in through the feed tube as well. It is important that the oil does not go in in a large splash. You should be pouring the oil in at a slow, but steady rate. It should resemble the thin stream of oil pictured above. As you near the end of the oil, you may pour a little faster.

5. When all the oil has been added, turn off the machine. The mayonnaise should be creamy, and a pale yellow color.

6. Store in a covered container, in the refrigerator.

FRESH AND FABULOUS GUACAMOLE

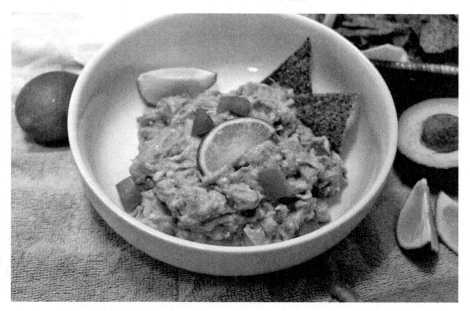

This guacamole has the vibrant flavors of avocados, tomatoes, and fresh lime juice. It makes a great dip for fresh veggies, and a nice sandwich spread, too. It's also wonderful served with chicken, fish, or fajitas.

Yield: 3 cups

Serving size: 1/4 cup

Ingredients:

» 2 very ripe avocados, mashed

- » 2 small tomatoes, chopped
- » 1/8 cup finely minced onion
- » 1 tsp fresh lemon juice
- » 2 tsp fresh lime juice
- » 1 tsp extra virgin olive oil
- » 3/4 tsp of dried cilantro or 2 tsp fresh
- » salt & pepper to taste

DIRECTIONS:

1. Mixing gently, combine all the ingredients in a medium bowl. Be careful not to over mix. Serve immediately.

2. To store leftovers, place the guacamole in an air tight container. Place an avocado pit in the center, cover tightly, and store in the refrigerator.

BABY SPINACH & BASIL PESTO

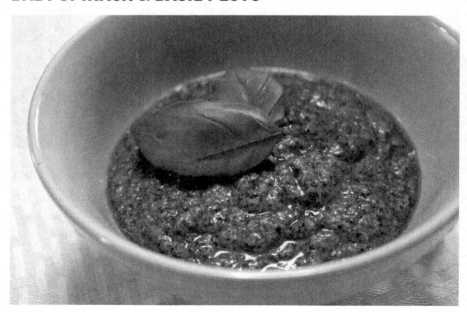

This bright flavored pesto makes a great topping for vegetables, fish, or lamb. It also works well as a dip for fresh vegetables, and as a zippy sandwich topping too.

Yield: 1 Cup

Serving Size: 1 Tbsp.

Ingredients:

» 1/2 cup fresh basil leaves, packed

» 1 1/2 cups fresh baby spinach leaves, packed

» 2 cloves of garlic

» 1/4 cup walnut pieces

» 2/3 cup extra virgin olive oil

» 1/2 cup grated parmesan cheese

» black pepper to taste

DIRECTIONS:

1. Place basil, spinach, garlic, and walnuts in the bowl of a food processor, fitted with a steel blade. Pulse until coarsely chopped.

2. With the processor on puree, slowly add the olive oil through the feed tube until the pesto is thoroughly pureed.

3. Add the parmesan and pepper, puree for 1 minute.

4. Serve immediately.

5. Store in the refrigerator or freezer, in a tightly covered container.

HEAVENLY HUMMUS – STAGE 3 ONLY

This hummus is so good, you'll be surprised by how quick and simple it is to make. Served with fresh cut up vegetables, it makes a great snack or party dip!

Yield: approx. 2.5 cups

Serving size: 2 tbsp.

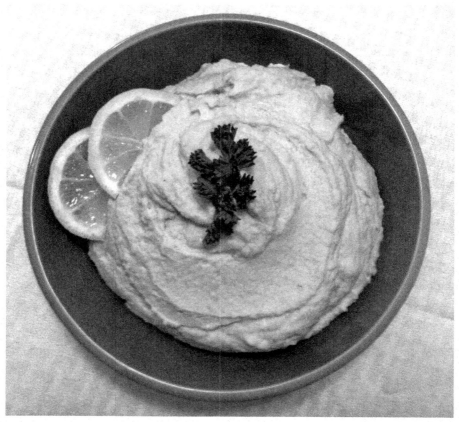

Ingredients:

- » 1 – 15 oz. can of organic garbanzo beans, rinsed and drained
- » 3 Tbsp. extra virgin olive oil
- » 1/4 cup all natural, organic tahini, (stir well before using)
- » 1/2 tsp garlic powder
- » 2 Tbsp. fresh lemon juice
- » approx. 3 Tbsp. cold filtered water
- » salt and pepper

DIRECTIONS:

1. Place the garbanzo beans, oil, tahini, garlic powder, lemon juice,

and water into a food processor fitted with a steel blade. Process until smooth, scraping down the sides of the bowl a few times. Depending on desired consistency, you may need to add 1-2 more tbsp. of water while processing.

2. Add salt and pepper to taste.

3. Store covered in a glass container, in the refrigerator. This hummus can be served immediately, but will taste even better the next day, after the flavors have blended together.

EASY WALNUT BUTTER

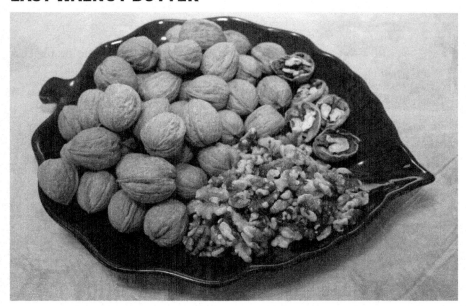

If you're a nut for walnuts, you're gonna love this recipe. Eat it with apple slices or carrot sticks for a snack, or use it as you would your favorite almond or peanut butter. The best part is how simple it is to make! You can have some ready to eat in under 15 minutes, and its taste gets even better after a day or two in the fridge.

Yield: 1 cup

Serving size: 2 tbsp.

Ingredients:

» 2 cups of walnut pieces

» 1/8 tsp of fine sea salt

» 4 tsp of walnut oil

DIRECTIONS:

1. Place nuts into a food processor that has been fitted with a steel blade. Grind the mixture (scraping it down as needed) for 2-3 minutes, or until it resembles a pastry flour that sticks together when you pinch it.

2. Add the salt.

3. While processing, gradually add in the oil. Continue to process until the walnuts bind together to form walnut butter.

4. Store in a closed container in the refrigerator.

CHOCOLATE WALNUT SPREAD – STAGE 3 ONLY

This chocolaty, dreamy spread is my walnutty version of Nutella. It's lovely with fresh fruit, such as strawberries or apple slices, for dessert. Spread on almond flour pancakes, it makes a special breakfast treat. It's so good, you can even use it as a creamy frosting.

Yield: approx. 2 cups

Serving size: 1 tbsp.

Added sugar per serving: 1 tsp.

Ingredients:

» 2 cups chopped walnuts

» 24 large, pitted dates

» a pinch of fine sea salt

» 1 1/2 tbsp. organic, 100% raw cacao powder

» 2 tsp walnut oil

» 1 scant cup of homemade coconut milk (recipe in breakfast section)

DIRECTIONS:

1. Place nuts and dates into a food processor that has been fitted with a steel blade. Grind the mixture (scraping it down as needed), for 2-3 minutes, or until it resembles a pastry flour that sticks together when you pinch it.

2. Add the cocoa powder and salt, processing to mix while adding the oil 1 tsp at a time.

3. Continue to process while gradually adding the coconut milk, and scraping the bowl down as needed. The finished product will be creamy, smooth, spreadable, and yummy!

4. Store in the refrigerator.

MAPLE WALNUT BUTTER – STAGE 3 ONLY

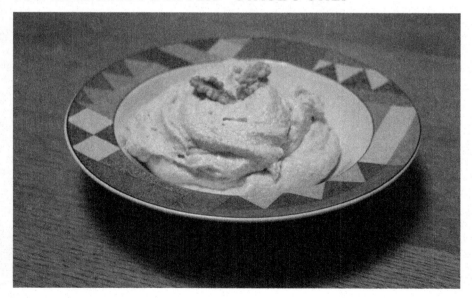

This silky maple walnut butter is nice when you're in the mood to indulge a little. It's great with strawberries, and other fresh fruit. It makes a decadent dessert topping, and a nice frosting, as well. For an extra special breakfast, spread some on the top of your pumpkin pancakes!

Yield: 1 cup

Serving size: 1 tbsp.

Added sugar per serving: ¾ tsp.

Ingredients:

» 2 cups walnut pieces

» 1/8 tsp fine sea salt

» 2 tsp walnut oil

» 4 tbsp. real maple syrup

» 1/2 tsp pure vanilla extract

» 1/2 cup water

DIRECTIONS:

1. Place the nuts into the bowl of a food processor that has been fitted with a steel blade. Grind the mixture (scraping it down as needed) for 2-3 minutes, or until it resembles a pastry flour that sticks together when you pinch it.

2. Add the salt.

3. While processing, gradually add in the oil, through the feed tube, until the butter is thoroughly combined.

4. Continue to process while gradually adding in the remaining ingredients.

5. The finished product will be a smooth spread, which is uniform in color and consistency.

MARINADES, & SALAD DRESSINGS

My favorite vinaigrette is very simple, and I use it all the time. It's just a squeeze of lemon juice, a good drizzle of olive oil, some salt, and some pepper. It's good on salads, and over vegetables. The flavor is bright and fresh. Below, I've included a few more structured recipes to help keep meals lively and interesting.

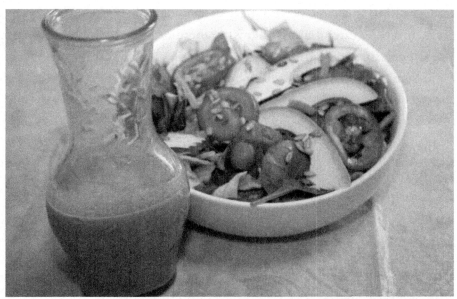

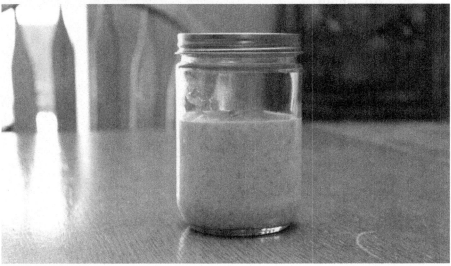

ZIPPY CHICKEN MARINADE

This marinade will make your chicken so incredibly flavorful, it's a no fail way to get rave reviews every time.

Just marinate chicken legs, thighs, wings, or breasts for a few hours in the refrigerator, then cook on the grill over a medium flame, or bake in the oven uncovered at 350°F, until cooked through.

To test for doneness, place a meat thermometer into the thickest part of the meat. Be careful not to allow the thermometer to touch the bone. The temperature on thermometer should climb quickly past 165°F. Check more than one piece of chicken to be sure they are all cooked evenly. The cooked chicken should not have any pink inside it, and the juices should run clear.

Ingredients:

- » The juice of 2 lemons
- » ½ cup of extra virgin olive oil
- » 6 cloves of garlic, minced or 1 tbsp. garlic powder
- » 1 tsp. sea salt
- » 2 tsp. black pepper
- » 2 tsp. cumin
- » 2 tsp. paprika
- » ½ tsp. turmeric
- » 1 tsp. dried parsley
- » A dash of cinnamon

DIRECTIONS:

1. Combine all the ingredients in a bowl. Mix well.
2. Arrange the chicken parts in a large baking dish.
3. Pour the marinade over the chicken.
4. Cover the baking dish with foil or plastic wrap. Refrigerate for at

least 1 hour.

5. Turn the chicken half way through the marinating time, to ensure even coverage.

6. Cook the chicken as described above.

BASIC VINAIGRETTE

This vinaigrette is good on salads or as a marinade for chicken or beef.

Yield: 1 cup

Ingredients

» 1/3 cup apple cider vinegar

» 2/3 cup extra virgin olive oil

» 1 clove of garlic

» 1 tsp fresh oregano

» 1 tsp fresh parsley

» 1/2 tsp sea salt

» 1/8 tsp black pepper

DIRECTIONS:

1. Place all the ingredients, except for the oil, into the bowl of a food processor that has been fitted with a steel blade.

2. Begin blending. While the processor is running, slowly pour the olive oil through the feed tube into the bowl.

3. Blend for a few seconds, until the dressing is thoroughly combined and becomes opaque.

RASPBERRY WALNUT VINAIGRETTE

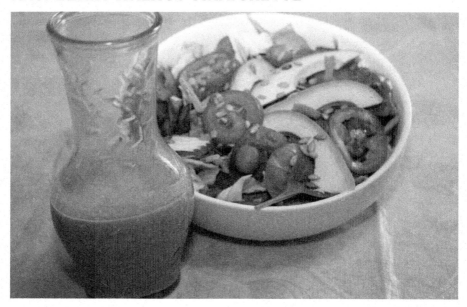

This one's great if you're in a hurry. It'll add some pizzazz to any salad, and works well as a marinade for poultry too.

Yield: 1 cup

Ingredients:

- » 6 Tbsp. walnut butter (find recipe under spreads)
- » 1/2 cup raspberry balsamic vinegar
- » 1/4 cup water

DIRECTIONS:

1. Add all the ingredients to a small bowl.
2. Whisk until emulsified.
3. Store in a covered container in the refrigerator. Shake well before serving.

BALSAMIC VINAIGRETTE

This dressing is nice on a salad, or poured over fresh vegetables.

- » 1/2 cup balsamic vinegar
- » 1 tsp fresh oregano
- » 1 tsp fresh parsley
- » 2/3 tsp fresh thyme
- » 1 clove of garlic
- » 1/4 tsp sea salt
- » 1/8 tsp black pepper
- » 2/3 cup extra virgin olive oil

Yield: 1 1/3 cups

DIRECTIONS:

1. Place all the ingredients, except for the olive oil, into the bowl of a food processor that has been fitted with a steel blade.

2. Begin blending. While the processor is running, slowly pour the olive oil through the feed tube into the bowl.

3. Blend for a few seconds, until the dressing is thoroughly combined and becomes opaque.

AVOCADO DRESSING

This dressing isn't at all sweet, but it is creamy, bold, and bursting with flavor. It's nice on salads, as a sauce for chicken or fish, and it makes a great dip for fresh veggies at snack time.

Yield: 2 cups

Ingredients:

- » 1 medium avocado, peeled & pitted
- » the juice of 1 fresh lemon
- » 1 cup of water

» 2 tbsp. extra virgin olive oil

» 1/2 tsp garlic powder

» 1 tsp onion powder

» 2 tbsp. dried cilantro/1 tbsp. fresh

» 1/4" piece of fresh turmeric, peeled

» 1 1/2 tsp paprika

» sea salt and black pepper to taste

DIRECTIONS:

1. Place all the ingredients into a high-speed blender, or into the bowl of a food processor that has been fitted with a steel blade.

2. Blend until smooth.

3. If the finished product is warm from processing, chill in the refrigerator before serving.

4. Store in a covered container under refrigeration.

QUICK RANCH DRESSING

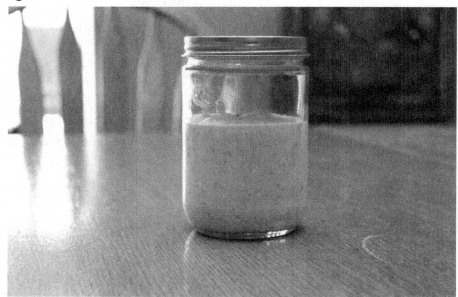

Here's a ranch dressing recipe that you can have ready for guests in under 10 minutes. I think you'll love the creamy, rich flavor. It'll taste even better if you have the time to let it refrigerate for an hour before serving.

Yield: 2 cups

Ingredients:

- » 1 cup cultured sour cream
- » 1/2 cup full fat Greek yogurt
- » 1 1/8 tsp apple cider vinegar
- » 2 tsp dried chives
- » 1 tsp dried parsley
- » 1/8 tsp mustard powder
- » 1 tsp garlic powder
- » 1/8 tsp celery seed
- » 2 tsp extra virgin olive oil
- » sea salt & black pepper to taste
- » filtered water

DIRECTIONS:

1. Place all the ingredients, except the water, into a large bowl and whisk until smooth.
2. Add salt and pepper to suit your taste.
3. Mix in 1/4 cup - 1/2 cup of water, to achieve desired consistency.
4. Store dressing in the refrigerator, in a covered jar or container.

QUICK CREAMY ITALIAN DRESSING

This is another great recipe for those special days when something creamy is in order.

Yield: 2 cups

- » 1 cup cultured sour cream
- » 1/2 cup full fat Greek yogurt
- » 1 1/8 tsp apple cider vinegar
- » 2 tbsp. grated parmesan
- » 2 tsp. dried parsley
- » ¾ tsp. garlic powder
- » ½ tsp. dried oregano
- » ½ tsp. onion powder
- » 1 tsp. dried basil
- » 4 tsp. extra virgin olive oil
- » 1 Dash paprika
- » sea salt & black pepper to taste
- » filtered water

DIRECTIONS:

1. Place all the ingredients, except the water, into a large bowl and whisk until smooth.
2. Add salt and pepper to suit your taste.
3. Mix in 1/4 cup - 1/2 cup of water, to achieve desired consistency.
4. Store dressing in the refrigerator, in a covered jar or container.

BAKED GOODS & DESSERTS

I prefer that your diet mainly consists of foods that are ingredients, instead of foods which are made from ingredients. That being said, I do understand that sometimes you're gonna want a slice of pizza, a burger on a bun, or a cookie, and that there are also special occasions, such as birthdays, anniversaries, holidays, and other social events that call for a special treat or dessert. I created this section of the book so that you can take part in all of life's holidays and celebrations without undermining your health. Just keep in mind that these recipes are more for now and then, and not for every meal or every day.

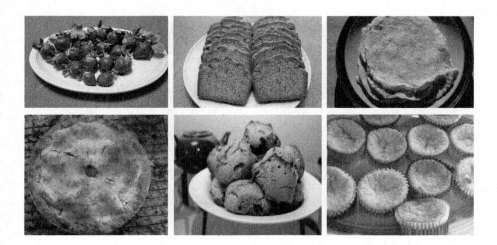

SANDWICH BREAD – STAGE 3 ONLY

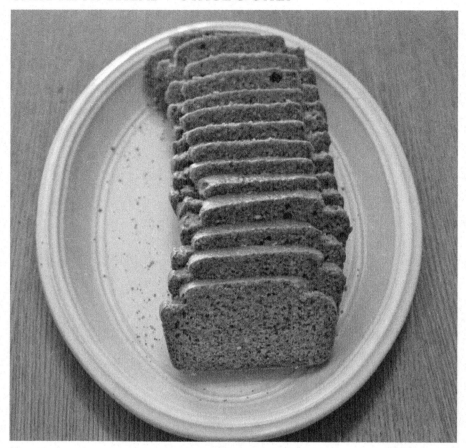

This bread is very easy to make. It's great for toasting and for sandwiches.

Yield: 1 loaf, (approx. 16 slices of bread)

Serving size: 2 slices

Added sugar per serving: 1/8 tsp.

Ingredients:

- » ½ cup almond meal/flour, packed
- » 1 tbsp. coconut flour
- » 1 tsp. aluminum free baking soda

- » ½ tsp. sea salt
- » 1 cup almond butter
- » 2 egg whites
- » 2 eggs
- » 1 tsp. organic raw honey
- » 1 tbsp. filtered water
- » 2 tsp. organic raw apple cider vinegar

DIRECTIONS:

1. Pre-heat the oven to 315 F
2. Grease a loaf pan.
3. Line the bottom of the loaf pan with parchment paper. Grease the paper.
4. Mix the dry ingredients in a small bowl.
5. Mix the wet ingredients in a medium sized bowl.
6. Add the dry ingredients into the wet ingredients, and mix well.
7. Pour the batter evenly into the prepared loaf pan.
8. Bake for 35-40 minutes, until a tooth pick inserted near the center comes out clean.
9. Cool in the pan for 10 minutes.
10. Remove from the pan, and cool on a wire rack until almost completely cool.
11. Place the loaf on a cutting board. Cut into slices, using a serrated bread knife.
12. Stagger the slices so they can finish cooling completely.
13. Store the completely cooled slices on a piece of paper toweling, inside an air tight container, in the refrigerator.

ARTISAN BREAD -STAGE 3 ONLY

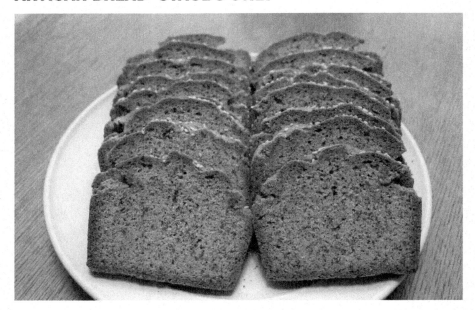

I make this bread all the time. The slices are a bit larger than the sandwich bread, it's delicious, and has a nice texture. It goes well with meals, it toasts great, and you can make sandwiches with it, too.

Yield: 1 loaf, (approx. 16 slices of bread)

Serving size: 2 slices

Added sugar per serving: 1/6 tsp.

Ingredients:

» 3 cups almond meal/flour, packed

» 3 tbsp. coconut flour

» 1 tbsp. aluminum free baking soda

» 4 ½ tbsp. flax meal

» ¾ tsp. sea salt

» 6 large eggs

» 3 tbsp. organic raw apple cider vinegar

» ¼ cup +1/8 cup almond butter

» 1 ½ tsp. organic raw honey

» 1 ½ tbsp. filtered water

» Optional: sesame seeds

DIRECTIONS:

1. Pre-heat the oven to 350°F

2. Grease a loaf pan.

3. Line the bottom of the loaf pan with parchment paper. Grease the paper.

4. Place all the dry ingredients into the bowl of a food processor that has been fitted with a steel blade. Pulse until well combined.

5. Add the wet ingredients to the bowl. Pulse until well combined.

6. Use a cake spatula to scoop the batter evenly into the prepared loaf pan.

7. Wet your hands under cold running water. Use your wet fingers to gently smooth the top of the bread into a loaf shape, and to smooth the dough to the edges of the pan.

8. Sprinkle the top with sesame seeds if desired.

9. Bake for 50-60 minutes, until a tooth pick inserted near the center comes out clean.

10. Cool in the pan for 10 minutes.

11. Remove from the pan, and cool on a wire rack until almost completely cool.

12. Place the loaf on a cutting board. Cut into slices, using a serrated bread knife.

13. Stagger the slices so they can finish cooling completely.

14. Store the completely cooled slices on a piece of paper toweling, inside an air tight container, in the refrigerator.

ARTISAN ROLLS – STAGE 3 ONLY

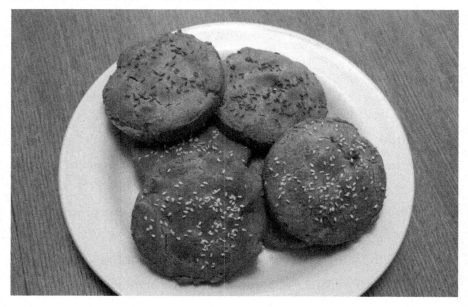

These rolls are the perfect size for burgers. They're so thick I sometimes cut them into thirds and toast them for sandwiches, but, then again, I used to cut my bagels into thirds, too. My husband likes to toast these rolls whole, and eat them with butter on them. Any way you slice them, though, they're great.

Yield: 6 rolls

Serving size: 1 roll

Added sugar per serving: 1/6 tsp.

Ingredients:

- » 2 cups almond meal/flour, packed
- » 2 tbsp. coconut flour
- » 2 tsp. aluminum free baking soda
- » 3 tbsp. flax meal
- » 1/2 tsp. sea salt
- » 4 large eggs

> » 2 tbsp. organic raw apple cider vinegar
> » ¼ cup almond butter
> » 1 tsp. organic raw honey
> » 1 tbsp. filtered water
> » Optional: sesame seeds

DIRECTIONS:

1. Pre-heat the oven to 350°F

2. Grease the cups of 2 large silicone, muffin top pans. Each pan should have 3 large muffin top cups. Place the silicone pans onto a large baking sheet or pizza pan, for support.

3. Place all the dry ingredients into the bowl of a food processor that has been fitted with a steel blade. Pulse until well combined.

4. Add the wet ingredients to the bowl. Pulse until well combined.

5. Use a cake spatula to scoop the batter evenly into the 6 prepared cups.

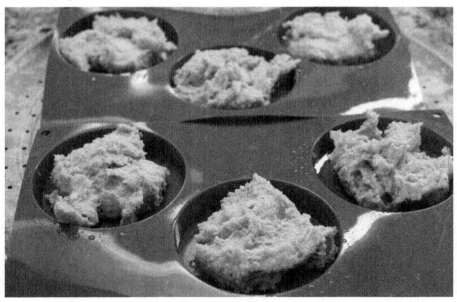

6. Wet your hands under cold running water. Use your wet fingers to gently smooth the dough to the edges of the muffin cups.

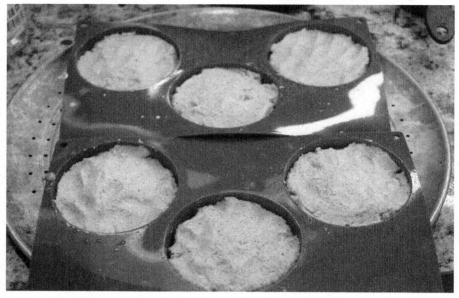

7. Sprinkle the tops with sesame seeds if desired.

8. Bake for 20-25 minutes, until a tooth pick inserted near the center comes out clean.

9. Cool in the pan for 10 minutes.

10. Carefully remove the rolls from the pan, and cool them on a wire rack until completely cool.

11. Store the completely cooled rolls on a piece of paper toweling, inside an air tight container, in the refrigerator.

ARTISAN GARLIC & ROSEMARY ROLLS -STAGE 3 ONLY

These are great with any meal, any time of the day.

Yield: 6 rolls

Serving size: 1 roll

Added sugar per serving: 1/6 tsp.

Ingredients:

- » 2 cups almond meal/flour, packed
- » 2 tbsp. coconut flour
- » 2 tsp. aluminum free baking soda
- » 3 tbsp. flax meal
- » 1/2 tsp. sea salt
- » ½ tbsp. garlic powder
- » 1 tbsp. dried rosemary
- » 1 tbsp. extra virgin olive oil
- » 4 large eggs
- » 2 tbsp. organic raw apple cider vinegar
- » ¼ cup almond butter
- » 1 tsp. organic raw honey
- » 1 tbsp. filtered water

DIRECTIONS:

1. Pre-heat the oven to 350°F

2. Grease the cups of 2 large silicone, muffin top pans. Each pan should have 3 large muffin top cups. Place the silicone pans onto a large baking sheet or pizza pan, for support.

3. Grind the rosemary into a fine powder, in a coffee grinder.

4. Place all the dry ingredients, including the rosemary, into the bowl of a food processor that has been fitted with a steel blade. Pulse until well combined.

5. Add the wet ingredients to the bowl. Pulse until well combined.

6. Use a cake spatula to scoop the batter evenly into the 6 prepared cups.

7. Wet your hands under cold running water. Use your wet fingers to gently smooth the dough to the edges of the muffin cups.

8. Bake for 20-25 minutes, until a tooth pick inserted near the center comes out clean.

9. Cool in the pan for 10 minutes.

10. Carefully remove the rolls from the pan, and cool them on a wire rack until completely cool.

11. Store the completely cooled rolls on a piece of paper toweling, inside an air tight container, in the refrigerator.

ARTISAN RYE ROLLS – STAGE 3 ONLY

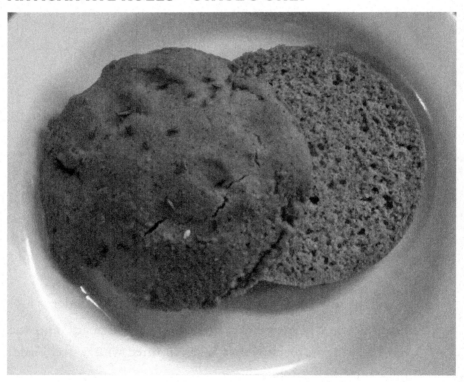

Make gourmet sandwiches by filling these rolls with smoked salmon, avocado slices, a slice of tomato and thinly sliced slivers of red onion.

Yield: 6 rolls

Serving size: 1 roll

Added sugar per serving: 1/6 tsp.

Ingredients:

» 2 cups almond meal/flour, packed

» 2 tbsp. coconut flour

» 2 tsp. aluminum free baking soda

» 3 tbsp. flax meal

» 2 tbsp. ground caraway seeds (grind in a coffee grinder)

» 1/2 tsp. sea salt

» 4 large eggs

» 2 tbsp. homemade coconut milk (recipe in breakfast section)

» 2 tbsp. organic raw apple cider vinegar

» ¼ cup almond butter

» 1 tsp. organic raw honey

» 1 tbsp. filtered water

» Optional: whole caraway seeds

DIRECTIONS:

1. Pre-heat the oven to 350°F

2. Grease the cups of 2 large silicone, muffin top pans. Each pan should have 3 large muffin top cups. Place the silicone pans onto a large baking sheet or pizza pan, for support.

3. Place all the dry ingredients into the bowl of a food processor that has been fitted with a steel blade. Pulse until well combined.

4. Add the wet ingredients to the bowl. Pulse until well combined.

5. Use a cake spatula to scoop the batter evenly into the 6 prepared cups.

6. Wet your hands under cold running water. Use your wet fingers to gently smooth the dough to the edges of the muffin cups.

7. Sprinkle the tops with whole caraway seeds, if desired.

8. Bake for 20-25 minutes, until a tooth pick inserted near the center comes out clean.

9. Cool in the pan for 10 minutes.

10. Carefully remove the rolls from the pan, and cool them on a wire rack.

11. Store the completely cooled rolls, on a piece of paper toweling, inside an air tight container, in the refrigerator.

ARTISAN ONION ROLLS – STAGE 3 ONLY

Because, onion rolls!

Yield: 6 rolls

Serving size: 1 roll

Added sugar per serving: 1/6 tsp.

Ingredients:

» 2 cups almond meal/flour, packed

» 2 tbsp. coconut flour

» 2 tsp. aluminum free baking soda

» 3 tbsp. flax meal

» 2 tbsp. dried minced onions

» 1/2 tsp. sea salt

» 4 large eggs

» 2 tbsp. organic raw apple cider vinegar

» ¼ cup almond butter

» 1 tsp. organic raw honey

» 1 tbsp. filtered water

» 2 tbsp. homemade coconut milk (recipe in breakfast section)

DIRECTIONS:

1. Pre-heat the oven to 350°F

2. Grease the cups of 2 large silicone, muffin top pans. Each pan should have 3 large muffin top cups. Place the silicone pans onto a large baking sheet or pizza pan, for support.

3. Place all the dry ingredients into the bowl of a food processor that has been fitted with a steel blade. Pulse until well combined.

4. Add the wet ingredients to the bowl. Pulse until well combined.

5. Use a cake spatula to scoop the batter evenly into the 6 prepared cups.

6. Wet your hands under cold running water. Use your wet fingers to gently smooth the dough to the edges of the muffin cups.

7. Sprinkle the tops with minced onion, if desired.

8. Bake for 20-25 minutes, until a tooth pick inserted near the center comes out clean.

9. Cool in the pan for 10 minutes.

10. Carefully remove the rolls from the pan, and cool them on a wire rack.

11. Store the completely cooled rolls on a piece of paper toweling, inside an air tight container, in the refrigerator.

BISCUITS – STAGE 3 ONLY

These biscuits remind me a lot of corn bread. They're moist and dense, and they pair wonderfully with soups and stews.

Yield: 12 biscuits

Ingredients:

» 2 cups almond meal/flour

» 2 cups garbanzo bean flour

» 4 tsp. aluminum free baking powder

» 1 tsp. sea salt

» ½ cup extra virgin olive oil

» 4 large eggs

» ½ cup homemade coconut milk (recipe in breakfast section)

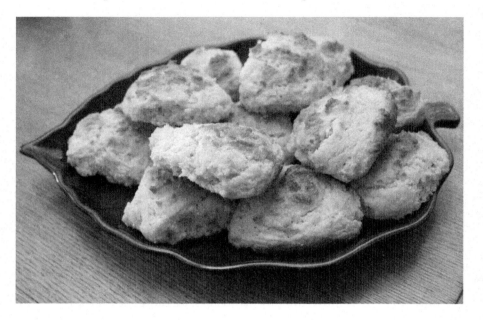

DIRECTIONS:

1. Pre-heat the oven to 400°F.

2. Place all the dry ingredients into the bowl of a food processor that has been fitted with a steel blade. Pulse until well combined.

3. Add the wet ingredients to the bowl. Pulse until well combined.

4. Let the dough rest for a few minutes.

5. While the dough is resting, grease two 8" cake pans, and line the bottoms with parchment paper.

6. Using a large ice cream scoop which has been dipped in cold water, place 6 large scoops of dough side by side in each pan, as pictured below.

7. Bake on the center rack of the pre-heated oven for 25 minutes, or until a tooth pick inserted near the center comes out clean.

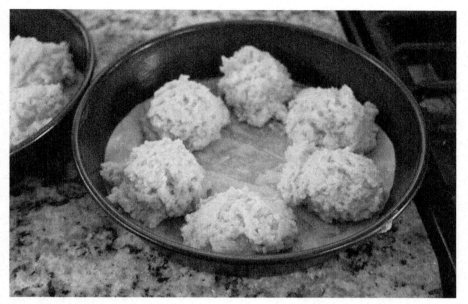

8. Cool in the pan for 10 minutes.

9. Carefully remove the biscuits from the pan, and cool them on a wire rack.

10. Store the cooled biscuits inside an air tight container, in the refrigerator.

CRÊPES

These crêpes are the perfect wrap for any of your favorite savory foods, from tuna salad to breakfast burritos, and more. You could also use them to make a sophisticated dessert by filling them with fresh warm berries, or chocolate walnut spread (recipe under spreads).

Yield: 6 crepes

Ingredients:

- » ¼ cup arrow root
- » ¼ cup coconut flour
- » 2 large eggs
- » Pinch of sea salt

» 1 cup homemade coconut milk (recipe in breakfast section)

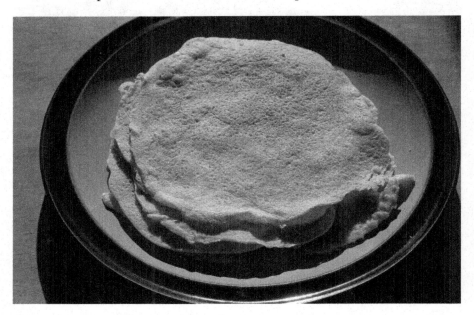

DIRECTIONS:

1. In a small bowl, combine the arrow root, the coconut flour, and the salt. Mix well with a fork.

2. In a larger bowl, whisk the eggs and the milk together until fluffy and well combined.

3. Whisk the dry ingredients into the egg mixture.

4. Grease a small sauté pan with butter, and heat over medium-low heat for a few seconds, to get it warmed up.

5. Pour about a ¼ cup of batter into the pan. Use the edge of a spatula to quickly spread the batter out to a thin pancake that is about 6" in diameter.

6. Cook for 2 full minutes.

7. Use the spatula to flip the crêpe over and cook for another 1-3 minutes. The crêpe should be lightly golden brown and crisp on both sides when done.

8. Repeat until all the batter is gone.

9. Serve immediately. Store leftovers in a covered container in the refrigerator.

TORTILLAS – STAGE 3 ONLY

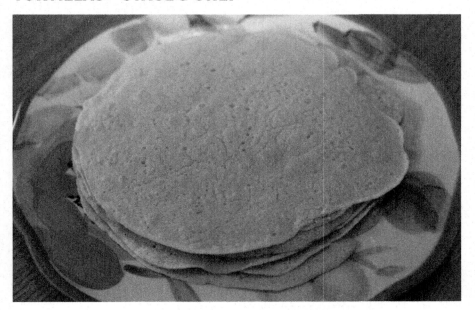

The texture and flavor of these tortillas go wonderfully with chili, fajitas, or your favorite Mexican fillings. They make good Quesadillas too.

Yield: 6 tortillas

Ingredients:

» 1 cup garbanzo bean flour

» 1 cup filtered water

» 2 tbsp. extra virgin olive oil

» A pinch of salt

DIRECTIONS:

1. In a bowl, whisk all the ingredients together.

2. Grease a small sauté pan with butter, and heat over medium-low heat for a few seconds, to get it warmed up.

3. Pour about a ¼ cup of batter into the pan. Swirl the pan to spread the batter into thin pancakes that are about 6" in diameter.

4. Cook until the edges dry, and you can see bubbles in the center.

5. Using a spatula, flip the tortilla and cook it for another 2 minutes. The finished tortilla should be lightly golden brown and crisp on both sides when done.

6. Serve immediately. Store leftovers in a covered container in the refrigerator.

SNACK CRACKERS – STAGE 3 ONLY

These little snack crackers are a healthy alternative to chips and pretzels, and they go well alongside soup or salad.

Yield: about 6 ½ dozen small crackers

Ingredients:

» 1 ½ cups almond meal/flour
» ½ cup garbanzo bean flour
» ½ cup coconut flour
» ½ cup grass-fed, salted butter
» 1 tsp. sea salt
» 2 large eggs
» Optional: 2-3 tsp. of sea salt, your favorite herbs and spices, or seeds.

DIRECTIONS:

1. Pre-heat the oven to 350°F.

2. Line a baking sheet with parchment paper.

3. Place all the ingredients into the bowl of a food processor that has

been fitted with a steel blade, and pulse until well combined and the dough forms a ball.

4. Divide the dough into 4 segments.

5. Place 1 segment between two large pieces of parchment paper. Use something heavy to weigh down the edges of the paper. Using a rolling pin, roll the dough out evenly, until it is about the same thickness as a thin cracker or a chip.

6. Remove the top piece of parchment paper. Using a pizza cutter, cut the dough into 1" squares. Remove any scraps of dough, and save them to reroll for more crackers.

7. Use a spatula to carefully transfer your crackers, one at a time, to the prepared baking sheet. Leave a ½" space between the crackers on the baking sheet.

8. Top with salt or herbs, spices, and seeds if desired, by sprinkling and pressing them onto the top of the crackers with your hands.

9. Place the baking sheet with the crackers onto the center rack of the pre-heated oven, and bake for 10 minutes.

10. After 10 minutes, remove the crackers from the oven and turn them over. Return them to the center rack of the oven, and bake them for another 5-8 minutes until they are crispy and light brown.

11. Remove the crackers from the oven and cool on a wire rack.

12. Repeat steps 5 – 10 with the remaining 3 segments of dough. Roll any scraps into the dough, until it has all been used.

13. Store the cooled crackers in a sealed container.

PIZZA

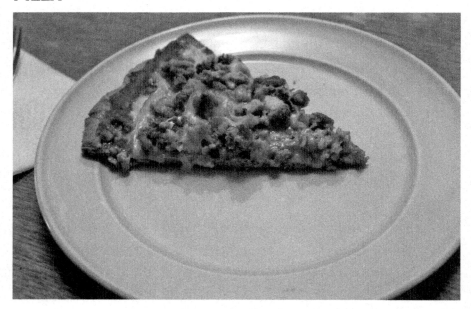

This pizza is very good. The edges are crispy, and each slice can stand up to a lot of extra toppings. So, on those days when it's pizza that you really want, enjoy!

Yield: 1 large pie

Dry Ingredients:

- » 2 cups almond meal
- » 2 tbsp. coconut flour
- » 1 tsp. aluminum free baking soda
- » 3 tbsp. flax meal
- » ½ tsp. salt
- » Optional: Italian seasoning to taste

Wet ingredients:

- » 4 eggs
- » 2 tbsp. organic raw apple cider vinegar
- » 1 tbsp. filtered water

» ¼ cup almond meal

Pizza Toppings:

» 6 oz. organic marinara sauce, with no added sugar

» 4-5 oz. mozzarella cheese & your favorite toppings

DIRECTIONS:

1. Pre-heat the oven to 350°F.

2. Cover a large pizza pan with parchment paper. Make sure that none of the paper is projecting out past the edge of the pan as it may burn.

3. Grease the parchment paper with extra virgin olive oil.

4. Place all the dry ingredients into the bowl of a food processor that has been fitted with a steel blade. Pulse until well combined.

5. Add the wet ingredients to the bowl. Pulse until well combined.

6. Using wet hands, spread the dough evenly over the prepared pizza pan to form a large pizza crust that is 1/8"-1/4" thick.

7. Place the crust onto the center rack of the preheated oven and bake for 25 minutes.

8. Remove the crust from the oven and allow it to cool for 5-10 minutes. Raise the oven temperature to 425°F.

9. While the crust is cooling, grate the mozzarella, and get your toppings ready.

10. Remove the parchment paper from underneath the crust. Top the crust with sauce, cheese, and toppings.

11. Return the pizza to the center rack of the oven, and bake for 10-15 minutes until the cheese is bubbly.

BLUEBERRY SCONES – STAGE 3 ONLY

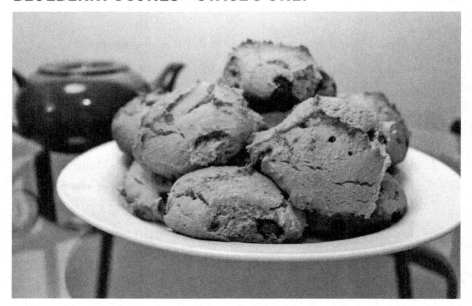

Yield: 12 scones

Serving size: 1 scone

Added sugar per serving: 1 tsp.

Ingredients:

> » 2 cups almond meal/flour
> » 2 cups garbanzo bean flour
> » 4 tsp. aluminum free baking powder
> » ¼ tsp. sea salt
> » ½ tsp. ground cinnamon
> » ½ cup extra virgin coconut oil
> » 4 large eggs
> » ½ cup homemade coconut milk (recipe in breakfast section)
> » 4 tbsp. organic raw honey
> » 1 ½ tsp. organic pure vanilla extract

» 1 cup fresh organic blueberries, rinsed and drained

DIRECTIONS:

1. Pre-heat the oven to 400°F.

2. Place all the dry ingredients into the bowl of a food processor that has been fitted with a steel blade. Pulse until well combined.

3. Add all the wet ingredients to the bowl, except for the berries. Pulse until well combined and smooth.

4. Using a cake spatula, scoop all the dough into a large bowl. Fold in the blueberries.

5. Let the dough rest for a few minutes.

6. While the dough is resting, grease two 8" cake pans, and line the bottoms with parchment paper.

7. Using a large ice cream scoop which has been dipped in cold water, place 6 large scoops of dough side by side in each pan.

8. Bake on the center rack of the pre-heated oven, for about 20 minutes, or until a tooth pick inserted near the center comes out clean.

9. Cool in the pan for 10 minutes.

10. Carefully, remove the scones from the pan, and cool them on a wire rack.

11. Store the cooled scones inside an air tight container, in the refrigerator.

GRANDMA'S COOKIES - STAGE 3 ONLY

These cookies are a revised version of a cookie recipe given to me by my grandmother. They come out soft, and taste a bit like an almond flavored macaroon. I think they're nice with a hot cup of tea.

Yield: 24 cookies

Serving size: 3 cookies

Added sugar per serving: 1 tsp.

Ingredients:

- » 2 large pastured eggs
- » ½ cup (8 tbsp.) grass fed, melted butter
- » 2 tsp. aluminum free baking powder
- » 1 tsp. vanilla
- » 2 cups almond meal/flour
- » 1 tbsp. coconut flour
- » 3 tbsp. honey
- » dash of cinnamon

DIRECTIONS:

1. Preheat the oven to 350°F.
2. Line a cookie sheet with parchment paper, and grease the surface.
3. Place all the ingredients into a large bowl and mix well to evenly combine.
4. Drop tablespoons of batter onto the cookie sheet, and flatten with the back of a fork. Space the cookies about ½" apart.
5. Place the cookie sheet with the cookies onto the center rack of the preheated oven, and bake for about 14 minutes, or until the cookies are lightly golden brown.

CHOCOLATE CHIP COOKIES - STAGE 3 ONLY

Yield: approximately 26-28 cookies

Serving size: 2 cookies

Added sugar per serving: 1 ½ tsp.

Ingredients:

- » 1 ½ cups almond flour
- » ½ cup garbanzo flour

- » ½ cup coconut flour
- » ½ cup (8 tbsp.) grass fed, salted butter
- » 1 tsp. pure vanilla extract
- » 2 large pastured eggs
- » 1/3 cup, plus 1 tbsp. organic coconut sugar
- » ½ tsp. cinnamon
- » 3 oz. 88% cacao chocolate, broken into small pieces
- » 1/3 cup walnut pieces

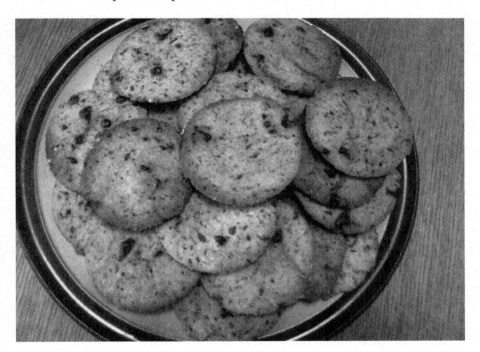

DIRECTIONS:

1. Preheat the oven to 350°F.
2. Line a baking sheet with parchment paper
3. Place all the ingredients, except for the chocolate and nuts, into the bowl of a food processor which has been fitted with a steel blade. Pulse until thoroughly combined.

4. Add the chocolate and nuts. Pulse lightly to just combine.

5. Divide the dough into 4 equal parts.

6. Roll out one section between two large pieces of parchment paper, to about 1/8"- ¼" thick. It is helpful to weigh the edges of the paper down with something heavy, to keep it from moving.

7. Cut into cookies, using a 2 ½" cookie cutter. Save any dough scraps for rerolling into more cookies.

8. Transfer the cookies onto the prepared baking sheet, using a metal spatula. Place the cookies about ½" apart.

9. When the cookie sheet is full, place it into the hot oven and bake for about 15 minutes, or until the cookies are lightly browned. Cool the baked cookies on a wire rack.

10. Repeat, until all the dough has been used up.

11. Store the cooled cookies in an air tight container.

CRUNCHY SESAME TEA BISCUITS – STAGE 3 ONLY

Yield: approximately 26-28 cookies

Serving size: 3 cookies

Added sugar per serving: 2 tsp.

Ingredients:

» 1 ½ cups almond flour

» ½ cup garbanzo flour

» ½ cup coconut flour

» ½ cup (8 tbsp.) grass fed, salted butter

» 1 tsp. pure vanilla extract

» 3 large pastured eggs

» 1/3 cup, plus 1 tbsp. organic coconut sugar

» 1 tsp. orange zest

» ½ tsp. cinnamon

» 1/8 tsp. nutmeg

» Sesame seeds

DIRECTIONS:

1. Preheat the oven to 350°F.

2. Line a baking sheet with parchment paper

3. Make an egg wash, by beating one of the eggs with 1 tsp. of the sugar, in a small bowl.

4. Set the egg wash on the side, and place the remaining ingredients, except for the sesame seeds, into the bowl of a food processor which has been fitted with a steel blade. Pulse until thoroughly combined.

5. Divide the dough into 4 equal parts.

6. Roll out one section, between two large pieces of parchment paper to about 1/8"- ¼" thick. It is helpful to weigh the edges of the paper down with something heavy, to keep it from moving.

7. Cut into cookies using a 2 ½" cookie cutter. Save any dough scraps for rerolling into more cookies.

8. Transfer the cookies onto the prepared baking sheet using a metal spatula. Place the cookies about ½" apart.

9. Brush each cookie with egg wash, and sprinkle with sesame seeds.

10. When the cookie sheet is full, place it into the hot oven and bake for about 15 minutes, or until the cookies are lightly browned. Cool the baked cookies on a wire rack.

11. Repeat until all the dough has been used up.

12. Store the cooled cookies in an air tight container.

HOLIDAY GINGERBREAD COOKIES – STAGE 3 ONLY

The winter holidays just wouldn't be the same without ginger bread cookies. These cookies capture both the spirit and the flavors of the season.

Yield: approximately 26-28 cookies

Serving size: 1 cookies

Added sugar per serving: 1 ½ tsp.

Ingredients:

  » 1 ½ cups almond flour

  » ½ cup garbanzo flour

  » ½ cup coconut flour

  » 1 pinch of salt

  » 2 tsp. powdered ginger

  » ½ cup grass-fed, butter

  » 2 large pastured eggs

  » 3tbsp. plus 2 tsp. organic coconut sugar

  » 3 tbsp. unsulfured molasses

DIRECTIONS:

1. Preheat the oven to 350°F.

2. Line a baking sheet with parchment paper

3. Place all the ingredients into the bowl of a food processor which has been fitted with a steel blade. Pulse until thoroughly combined.

4. Divide the dough into 4 equal parts.

5. Roll out one section between two large pieces of parchment paper, to about 1/8"- ¼" thick. It is helpful to weigh the edges of the paper down with something heavy, to keep it from moving.

6. Cut into cookies using a 2 ½" cookie cutter.

7. Transfer the cookies onto the prepared baking sheet using a metal spatula. Place the cookies about ½" apart.

8. When the cookie sheet is full, place it into the hot oven and bake for about 15 minutes, or until the cookies are lightly browned.

Cool the baked cookies on a wire rack.

9. Repeat, until all the dough has been used up.

10. Store the cooled cookies in an air tight container.

CHOCOLATE HAZELNUT COOKIES – STAGE 3 ONLY

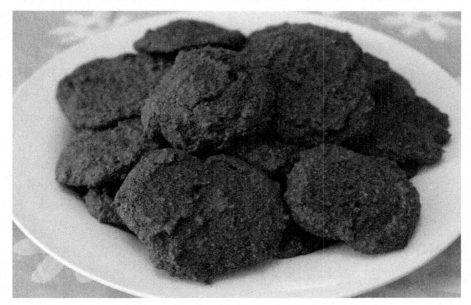

These cookies are my daughters favorite.

Yield: 24 cookies

Serving size: 4 cookies

Added sugar per serving: 2 tsp.

Ingredients:

- » 2 large pastured eggs
- » ½ cup softened, grass-fed butter
- » 2 tsp. aluminum free baking soda
- » 1 tsp. vanilla
- » 2 cups hazelnut flour
- » 1 tbsp. coconut flour

>> 3 ½ tbsp. honey

>> dash of cinnamon

>> pinch of salt

DIRECTIONS:

1. Preheat the oven to 320 F.

2. Line a cookie sheet with parchment paper, and grease the surface.

3. Place all the ingredients into a large bowl, and mix well to evenly combine.

4. Drop tablespoons of batter onto the cookie sheet, and flatten with the back of a fork. Space the cookies about ½" apart.

5. Place the cookie sheet with the cookies, onto the center rack of the preheated oven, and bake for about 15 minutes, or until the cookies are done.

ALMOND FINGERS – STAGE 3 ONLY

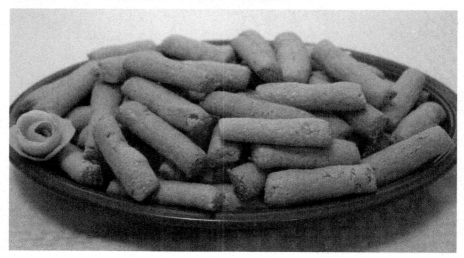

You'll find the rich taste of almonds to be in perfect harmony with the bright taste of fresh lemon peel, in these elegant finger-sized cookies. They're a takeoff on the biscuit like cookies my grandmother used to bake when I was a child. Making them always makes me think of her, and brings a smile to my face. The sweet fragrance of them baking is wonderful. I love the fact that they are so low in sugar, and of course they contain all the healthy benefits that you get from eating almonds like, being good for your heart and lowering your risks for getting cancer.

Yield: 72 cookies

Serving size: 2 cookies

Added sugar per serving: 1 tsp.

Ingredients:

- » 2 large pastured eggs
- » 4 large pastured egg whites
- » 3/4 cup organic coconut sugar
- » 1/2 cup melted butter
- » 2 tsp. pure vanilla extract
- » 6 1/2 cups of finely ground almond flour
- » 4 tsp. baking powder
- » 2 tsp. fresh lemon zest, finely grated or minced

DIRECTIONS:

1. Preheat the oven to 300 degrees F.

2. In a large bowl, beat the eggs and egg whites until they are fluffy. Reserve about 4 Tbsp. of egg mixture in a small bowl or cup.

3. To the large bowl, add the sugar, melted butter, and vanilla, beating well after each addition.

4. In a medium bowl, combine the flour, lemon zest, and baking powder. Mix well, with a fork or a whisk, until they are completely incorporated.

5. Mixing well, slowly add the dry mixture in small increments to the egg mixture. When the dough is ready, it will be slightly sticky

but easy to roll.

6. On a clean, unfloured surface, roll the dough out into ropes that are approximately 1/2 " thick. Using a knife or a pizza cutter, cut the rope into 3" lengths.

7. Place the cookies on to an ungreased cookie sheet. Space the cookies about a 1/2" apart.

8. Bake the cookies on the center rack of the oven for about 20 minutes, or until the bottoms are golden brown and the tops are starting to brown a bit as well.

9. Cool on a wire rack.

10. Store the cooled cookies in a covered container, at room temperature.

BROWNIES – STAGE 3 ONLY

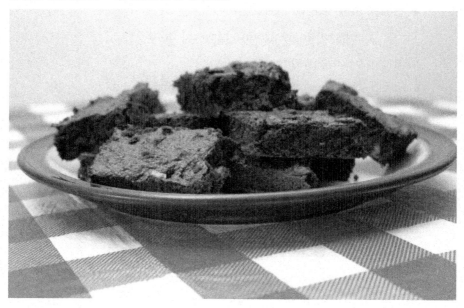

These brownies come out fudgy and moist. They are so good, people would never know that they weren't made with white flour.

Yield: 14 brownies

Serving size: 1 brownie

Added sugar per serving: 2/3 tsp.

Ingredients:

- » 1/8 cup coconut flour
- » ¾ cup almond meal/flour
- » 1/3 cup chopped walnuts
- » ½ tsp. aluminum free baking soda
- » Pinch of salt
- » 6 oz. of 88% cacao chocolate, chopped or broken into small pieces
- » ¼ cup organic, extra virgin coconut oil
- » ½ tsp. pure vanilla extract
- » 1 banana, mashed
- » 2 large eggs

DIRECTIONS:

1. Preheat the oven to 320 F.
2. Grease an 8" pan with coconut oil, or butter.
3. Place the flours, walnuts, baking soda, and salt into a bowl. Use a wire whisk to combine these ingredients.
4. Create a double boiler by filling a small sauce pan about 1/3 of the way full with water, and placing a large metal bowl on top of the pan. The bottom of the bowl should sit about 1/3 of the way down into the pan.
5. Place the pan with the bowl onto the stove over a medium-low heat.
6. Place the chocolate, and the oil into the bowl. Mix constantly, until the chocolate has completely melted and is smooth. Remove from the heat.

7. Using a spoon, beat the dry ingredients, the vanilla, and the mashed banana into the chocolate mixture.

8. Beat in the eggs.

9. Evenly spread the batter into the prepared pan.

10. Place the pan onto the center rack of the preheated oven. Bake for about 30 minutes or until a tooth pick inserted near the center comes out clean.

11. Cool completely on a wire rack.

12. Cut the brownies into 14 two inch squares. Store the brownies in a covered container.

LEMON CUPCAKES – STAGE 3 ONLY

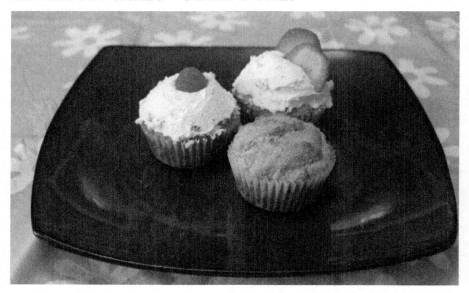

These moist, lemony cupcakes are great for special occasions. I made them for my Mother's 77th birthday. I frosted them with my lemon frosting recipe (in this section), and she absolutely loved them. Since the cupcake recipes contain 2 tsp. of added sugar each, if you would like to eat them frosted you will have to cut back on your dark chocolate for the day accordingly.

Yield: 9 cupcakes

Serving size: 1 cupcake

Added sugar per serving: 2 tsp.

Ingredients:

- » 2 1/8 cups almond meal/flour
- » 1 tsp. aluminum free baking powder
- » Pinch sea salt
- » Zest of one lemon, minced
- » 8 tbsp. grass fed-butter, softened
- » 1/3 cup organic coconut sugar
- » 1 tsp. organic raw honey
- » 1 tsp. pure vanilla extract
- » 3 large pastured eggs
- » 2 tbsp. fresh lemon juice
- » 2 tbsp. water

DIRECTIONS:

1. Preheat the oven to 350°F.

2. Line the cups of a standard cupcake pan, with paper liners.

3. Place the almond meal, baking powder, salt, and lemon zest into a large bowl. Whisk to combine.

4. In a small bowl, cream the butter and the sugar together.

5. Add the remaining ingredients to the butter mixture one at a time, whisking well after each addition.

6. Add the butter and egg mixture, to the almond meal mixture in the large bowl. Whisk until the batter is smooth.

7. Spoon the batter evenly into the prepared pan to make 9 cupcakes.

8. Place the pan onto the center rack of the preheated oven and bake for approximately 25 minutes, or until a tooth pick inserted near the middle of a cupcake comes out dry, and the cupcakes spring back gently when pressed lightly.

9. Cool on a wire rack.

10. When completely cool, frost each cupcake with 1 tbsp. of lemon frosting, if desired.

11. Store in an airtight container, in the refrigerator.

CAPPUCCINO CUPCAKES – STAGE 3 ONLY

These are for the adults, but I bet the kids will love them too! Since the cupcake recipes contain 2 tsp. of added sugar each, if you would like to eat them frosted you will have to cut back on your dark chocolate for the day accordingly.

Yield: 9 cupcakes

Serving size: 1 cupcake

Added sugar per serving: 2 tsp.

Ingredients:

» 1 ½ cups almond meal/flour

» 6 tbsp. raw 100% cacao powder

» 1 tbsp. cinnamon

» 1 tsp. aluminum free baking powder

» pinch of sea salt

» 8 tbsp. grass-fed butter, softened

» 1/3 cup organic coconut sugar

» 1 tsp. organic raw honey

» 1 tsp. vanilla

» 3 large pastured eggs

» 1 tsp. organic raw apple cider vinegar

» 2 tbsp. cold coffee

DIRECTIONS:

1. Preheat the oven to 350°F.

2. Line the cups of a standard cupcake pan, with paper liners.

3. Place the almond meal, baking powder, salt, cacao powder and cinnamon, into a large bowl. Whisk to combine.

4. In a small bowl, cream the butter and the sugar together.

5. Add the remaining ingredients to the butter mixture one at a time, whisking well after each addition.

6. Add the butter and egg mixture, to the almond meal mixture in the large bowl. Whisk until the batter is smooth.

7. Spoon the batter evenly into the prepared pan to make 9 cupcakes.

8. Place the pan onto the center rack of the preheated oven, and bake for approximately 25. Minutes, or until a tooth pick inserted near the middle of a cupcake comes out dry, and the cupcakes spring back gently when pressed lightly.

9. Cool on a wire rack.

10. When completely cooled, frost each cupcake with 1 tbsp. of tiramisu flavored, mascarpone cheese, if desired.

11. Store in an airtight container, in the refrigerator.

YELLOW CUPCAKES – STAGE 3 ONLY

Since the cupcake recipes contain 2 tsp. of added sugar each, if you would like to eat them frosted you will have to cut back on your dark chocolate for the day accordingly.

Yield: 9 cupcakes

Serving size: 1 cupcake

Added sugar per serving: 2 tsp.

Ingredients:

- » 2 1/8 cups almond meal/flour
- » 1 tsp. aluminum free baking powder
- » pinch sea salt
- » zest of one orange, minced
- » 8 tbsp. grass fed-butter, softened
- » 1/3 cup organic coconut sugar
- » 1 tsp. organic raw honey
- » 1 tsp. pure vanilla extract
- » 3 large pastured eggs
- » 2 tbsp. fresh orange juice
- » 2 tbsp. water

DIRECTIONS:

1. Preheat the oven to 350°F.
2. Line the cups of a standard cupcake pan, with paper liners.
3. Place the almond meal, baking powder, salt, and orange zest into a large bowl. Whisk to combine.
4. In a small bowl, cream the butter and the sugar together.
5. Add the remaining ingredients to the butter mixture one at a time, whisking well after each addition.
6. Add the butter and egg mixture to the almond meal mixture in the large bowl. Whisk until the batter is smooth.
7. Spoon the batter evenly into the prepared pan to make 9 cupcakes.
8. Place the pan onto the center rack of the preheated oven, and bake for approximately 25. Minutes, or until a tooth pick inserted near the middle of a cupcake comes out dry, and the cupcakes

spring back gently when pressed lightly.

9. Cool on a wire rack.

10. When completely cool, frost each cupcake with 1 tbsp. of vanilla frosting, if desired.

11. Store in an airtight container, in the refrigerator.

LEMON FROSTING – STAGE 3 ONLY

Yield: 2 cups

Serving size: 2 tbsp.

Added sugar per serving: 2/3 tsp.

Ingredients:

- » 8 oz. mascarpone cheese
- » 4 oz. cream cheese, softened
- » 2 tbsp. lemon juice
- » 2 tbsp. organic raw honey
- » ¾ tsp. vanilla
- » 1 ½ tbsp. organic coconut sugar
- » 2 tbsp. sour cream

DIRECTIONS:

1. Place all the ingredients into a medium sized bowl.

2. Using an electric hand mixer, beat together until creamy, glossy, and smooth.

3. Store any leftovers in a covered container in the refrigerator.

VANILLA FROSTING – STAGE 3 ONLY

Yield: 1 1/3 cups

Serving size: 2 tbsp.

Added sugar per serving: ¼ tsp.

Ingredients:

- » 1 cup mascarpone cheese
- » 1 tbsp. fresh orange juice
- » 2 ½ tsp. organic raw honey
- » 1 tsp. vanilla

DIRECTIONS:

1. Place all the ingredients into a medium sized bowl.
2. Using an electric hand mixer, beat together until creamy, glossy, and smooth.
3. Store any leftovers in a covered container in the refrigerator.

CHEESE CAKE BITES – STAGE 3 ONLY

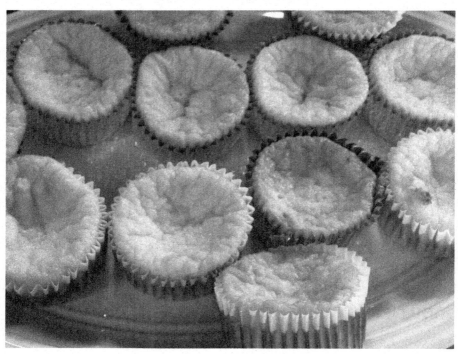

Yield: 12 Cheese cake bites

Serving Size: 1 Cheese cake bite

Added sugar per serving: 1 ¼ tsp.

Ingredients:

- » 2 large pastured eggs
- » 1/3 cup organic raw honey
- » ¼ tsp. salt
- » 15 oz. whole milk ricotta cheese
- » 4 oz. cream cheese, softened
- » 1 tsp. orange/lemon zest, minced
- » ½ tsp. vanilla

DIRECTIONS:

1. Preheat the oven to 350°F.
2. Line a standard 12 cup, cupcake pan with paper cupcake liners.
3. In a large bowl, whisk the eggs, honey, and salt till foamy.
4. Add the remaining ingredients, and whisk till smooth.
5. Pour the batter into the prepared pan, distributing it evenly between the 12 cups.
6. Place the pan onto the center rack of the preheated oven, and bake for 25-30 minutes, or until the bites are set, and lightly golden brown.
7. Cool on a wire rack. Store in a covered container in the refrigerator.

MINI PUMPKIN PIES – STAGE 3 ONLY

Yield: 12 tartlets

Serving size: 1 tartlet

Added sugar per serving: 1 ¾ tsp.

Ingredients for pie filling:

» 1 cup organic pumpkin puree

» 1 cup homemade coconut milk (recipe in this breakfast section)

» ½ tsp. sea salt

» 1/3 cup organic coconut sugar + 2 tbsp.

» 1 tsp. ground cinnamon

» 1 tsp. ground ginger

» ½ tsp. allspice

» 2 large pastured eggs.

Ingredients for the tartlets:

» ¾ cup almond flour

» ¼ cup garbanzo bean flour

» ¼ cup coconut flour

» ¼ cup salted, grass fed butter

» 1 large pastured egg

DIRECTIONS:

1. Preheat the oven to 350°F.

2. Line a standard 12 cup, cupcake pan with paper cupcake liners.

3. Combine all the ingredients for the filling in a bowl. Mix well.

4. Place the filling into the refrigerator, while you prepare the dough for the tartlets.

5. Place all the ingredients for the tartlets, into the bowl of a food processor that has been fitted with a steel blade.

6. Pulse until the dough pulls away from the sides of the bowl and forms a ball.

7. Divide the dough into 2 parts.

8. Place ½ of the dough between two large sheets of parchment paper. Weigh down the ends of the paper, and roll the dough out

until it is about 1/8"-1/4 "thick.

9. Use a round 2 ½" cookie cutter, to cut the dough into circles.

10. Gently push 1 dough circle into the bottom of a cupcake liner. Use your fingers to gently even out and press together any dough that separates in the liner. Save any dough scraps for rerolling.

11. Repeat until you have used up all the dough. You should have 12 tartlets when you are done.

12. Place the pan with the tartlets, onto the center rack of the pre-heated oven, and bake for 15 minutes.

13. Remove them from the oven, and allow them to cool for 2-3 minutes.

14. Take the filling out of the refrigerator. Stir it once or twice to make sure it is fully incorporated.

15. Spoon equal amounts of filling into the baked tartlets.

16. Return the pan to the oven, and bake until the centers of the mini pies have set.

17. Cool on a wire rack. Store fully cooled pies in the refrigerator, in a covered container.

APPLE CRUMBLE – STAGE 3 ONLY

Yield: 8 servings

Serving size: 1 portion

Added sugar per serving: 1 ½ tsp.

Ingredients:

» 4 tbsp. organic coconut sugar divided, evenly

» 6 Apples, peeled, cored, and sliced

» 1 2/3 tbsp. arrow root

» ¼ tsp. ground cinnamon + extra for filling

» ground ginger

» ¼ cup hazelnut flour

» ¼ cup almond meal

» 1 tbsp. grass fed butter

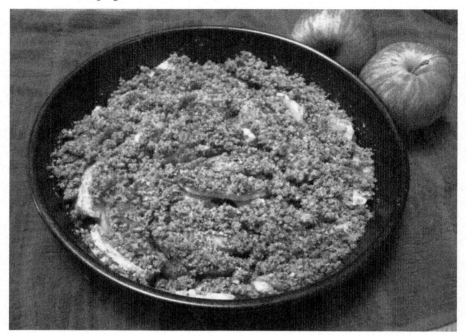

DIRECTIONS:

1. Preheat the oven to 350°F.

2. Grease an 8" cake pan.

3. Place 2 tbsp. of sugar on the side to be reserved for the topping.

4. Place a single layer of apples on the bottom of the pan.

5. Sprinkle the apples with a little sugar, cinnamon, ginger, and arrow root.

6. Keep layering the apples, sprinkling each layer with sugar, cinnamon, ginger, and arrow root, until all the apples have been used.

7. In a small bowl, mix together the remaining 2tbsps. of sugar, ¼ tsp. of cinnamon, and the nut flours.

8. Add the butter to the bowl. Use your fingers to combine the butter and flour mixture, until it has the texture of wet sand.

9. Sprinkle the topping over the apples in the pan.

10. Place the crumble onto the center rack of the preheated oven.

11. Bake for 60-70 minutes until the apples are tender.

12. Serve warm or cool on a wire rack.

13. Store leftovers covered, in the refrigerator.

PEACH COBBLER – STAGE 3 ONLY

Yield: 8 slices

Serving size: 1 slice

Added sugar per serving: 1 ½ tsp.

Ingredients for the crust:

- » 2 large pastured eggs
- » ½ cup/8 tbsp. grass fed, melted butter
- » 2 tsp. aluminum free baking powder
- » 1 tsp. vanilla
- » 2 cups almond meal/flour
- » 1 tbsp. coconut flour
- » 2 tbsp. honey
- » dash of cinnamon

Ingredients for the filling:

- » 12oz. frozen peaches
- » ½ tsp. ground cinnamon
- » 1/8 tsp. ground ginger
- » 1 tbsp. organic coconut sugar
- » 1 tbsp. organic, raw honey

DIRECTIONS:

1. Preheat the oven to 350°F.

2. Grease an 8" cake pan with coconut oil or butter.

3. Place all the ingredients for the crust into a bowl. Mix well to incorporate into a dough.

4. Reserve 1/3 of this mixture for the topping.

5. Taking small handfuls of the remaining 2/3's of the dough, line the cake pan.

6. Use your fingers to gently press the dough into the bottom, and up the sides of the pan. When you're finished, the dough should extend an inch or so, past the edge of the pan.

7. In a separate bowl, combine all the ingredients for the filling, and toss well.

8. Pour the filling evenly into the prepared crust.

9. Fold the extended edges of the dough over the filling.

10. Dot the top of the cobbler with the reserved 1/3 of the dough.

11. Sprinkle the top with additional cinnamon, if desired, and place it onto the center rack of the preheated oven.

12. Bake the cobbler for 35 minutes or the fruit is tender and the crust is golden brown.

13. Cool on a wire rack. Store the cooled cobbler covered, in the refrigerator.

FRUIT PIE – STAGE 3 ONLY

Make a delicious fruit pie for dessert on the holidays, using this easy recipe.

Yield: 8 servings

Serving size: 1 slice

Added sugar per serving: 1 ½ tsp.

Ingredients for the pie crust:

- » 1 ½ cups almond flour
- » ½ cup garbanzo bean flour
- » ½ cup coconut flour
- » ½ cup salted grass-fed butter
- » 1 tsp. sea salt
- » 2 large pastured eggs + 1 egg for egg wash
- » ½ tsp. organic coconut sugar

Ingredients for fruit filling:

- » 5 cups of fresh or frozen fruit
- » 1 tbsp. & ½ tsp. of organic coconut sugar
- » 2 tsp. arrow root powder
- » ground cinnamon
- » ground ginger

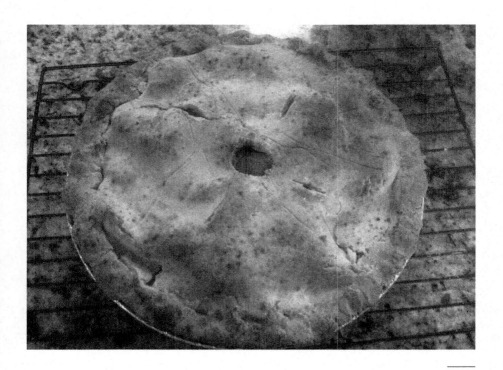

DIRECTIONS:

1. Preheat the oven to 350°F.

2. Grease an 8" pie tin with coconut oil or butter.

3. To make the crust, place the flours, butter, salt, and 2 of the eggs, into the bowl of a food processor which has been fitted with a steel blade. (Save the remaining egg and ½ tsp. of sugar on the side, they will be used to glaze the top crust before baking the pie.)

4. Pulse until the dough pulls away from the sides of the bowl, and forms a ball.

5. Divide the dough into equal 2 parts. Completely wrap ½ of the dough with parchment paper, and place it into the refrigerator.

6. Place the other ½ of the dough between two large sheets of parchment paper. Weigh down the ends of the paper, and roll the dough out into a circle is of even thickness, which is slightly larger than the pie tin.

7. Remove the top piece of parchment, and carefully invert the dough into the pie tin.

8. Use your fingers to gently press the dough into the tin, and to even out the dough.

9. Trim any excess dough from the edges of the pie tin, and use them to patch the crust in any areas that might need filling in.

10. Place the pie tin onto the center rack of the preheated oven, and bake it for 15-20 minutes, or until the edges just begin to turn golden brown.

11. Remove the bottom crust from the oven.

12. To fill the crust, Place a single layer of fruit on the bottom of the crust.

13. Sprinkle the fruit with a little sugar, cinnamon, ginger, and arrow root.

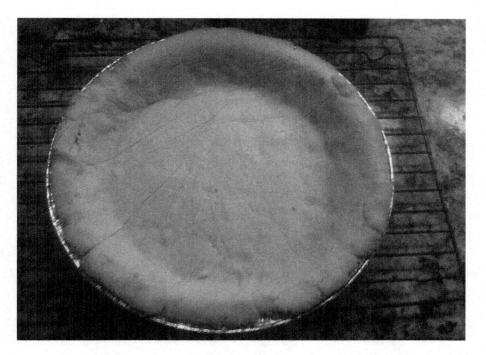

14. Keep layering fruit, sugar, cinnamon, ginger, and arrow root, until all the filling ingredients have been used up, heaping the fruit towards the center as you go.

15. Take the remaining ½ of the dough out of the refrigerator.

16. Place it between two large sheets of parchment paper. Weigh down the ends of the paper, and roll the dough out into a circle is of even thickness, which is slightly larger than the pie tin.

17. Remove the top piece of parchment, and carefully invert the dough onto the top of the pie.

18. Trim any excess dough from the edges of the pie tin, and use it to patch the crust in any areas that might need filling in, especially around the edges.

19. Using your fingers gently press the edges of the pie crust together.

20. Using a fork, or your fingers, pinch the edges of the crust together to make the decorative edge.

21. Use a small sharp knife to cut a vent hole in the center of the top of the pie crust. Use the same knife to make 4 small, 1" slashes in the top of pie crust. (The vent hole, and slashes, are made to allow steam to escape during the baking process.)

22. In a small bowl, beat the remaining egg.

23. Brush the top of the crust with the egg, and sprinkle it with the reserved ½ tsp. of sugar.

24. Bake the pie on the center rack of the preheated oven for about 1 hour, or until the fruit is tender and the crust is golden brown.

25. Cool on a wire rack. Store leftovers covered in the refrigerator.

CHERRY CHEESE CAKE – STAGE 3 ONLY

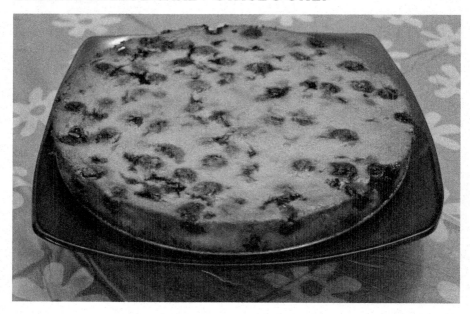

This dessert is perfect for a really special occasion, like Valentine's day, or an anniversary dinner.

Yield: 10 servings

Serving size: one slice

Added sugar per serving: 1 ½ tsp.

Ingredients for the crust:

» ½ cup almond meal

» 1 cup chopped walnuts

» 1 tbsp. organic extra virgin coconut oil

Ingredients for cake:

» 3 ½ cups frozen dark cherries

» 1 tbsp. arrow root powder

» 2 large pastured eggs

» 1/3 cup organic raw honey

» ¼ tsp. sea salt

» 15 oz. whole milk ricotta cheese

» 4 oz. cream cheese, softened

» 1 tsp. of orange or lemon zest

» ½ tsp. pure vanilla extract

DIRECTIONS:

1. Preheat the oven to 350° F.

2. Grease a 10" spring form pan.

3. Place the ingredients for the crust into a small bowl. Using your fingers, or a fork, mix the ingredients thoroughly, until the texture is that of wet sand.

4. Press the nut mixture, evenly, onto the bottom of the prepared spring form pan.

5. In another bowl, toss the cherries with the arrow root powder.

6. Distribute the cherries evenly over the crust.

7. In a larger, clean bowl combine the eggs, honey, and salt. Whisk until foamy.

8. Add in the ricotta, cream cheese, vanilla, and zest. Whisk again,

until well incorporated and smooth.

9. Pour the cheese mixture evenly over the cherries.

10. Place the pan onto the center rack of the preheated oven.

11. Bake for approximately 1 ½ hours, or until the center is set and the edges begin to turn golden brown.

12. Cool on a wire rack for about 15 minutes.

13. After 15 minutes remove the collar from the spring form pan. Continue cooling on the wire rack, until the cake is completely cool.

14. Store the cooled cake, covered in the refrigerator.

CHOCOLATE COVERED STRAWBERRIES

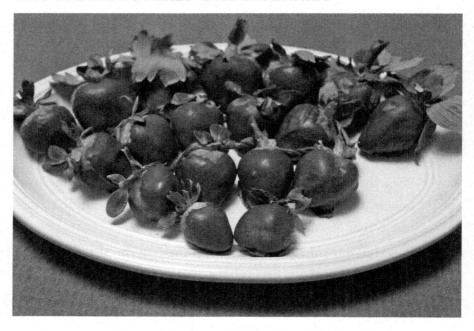

The quintessential romantic treat for that special someone, on that special day. Six berries are equivalent to the allotted 1 ounce of dark chocolate per day, so this is a treat you can opt for any day that you like!

Yield: about 18 large strawberries

Serving size: 6 berries

Ingredients:

- » 1 lb. large ripe organic strawberries
- » ¼ cup of full fat, canned, organic coconut milk
- » 2 ¼ tsp organic, extra virgin coconut oil or grass-fed butter
- » 3 oz. of 72% cacao dark chocolate, chopped up or broken into small pieces

DIRECTIONS:

1. Rinse the strawberries, and pat them dry with paper toweling.
2. Line a baking sheet with parchment paper.
3. Place the chopped chocolate into a bowl.
4. Place the milk and oil into a sauce pan. Warm the milk mixture over a medium heat until it begins to bubble around the edges, but do not allow it to come to a boil.
5. Pour the heated milk mixture over the chocolate in the bowl and mix constantly, until all the chocolate has melted and is smooth.
6. Holding the berries by their green tops, dip them one by one into the chocolate and place them onto the prepared baking sheet.
7. When all the berries have been dipped into chocolate, place the baking sheet full of berries into the refrigerator to harden for an hour or two.
8. Once the chocolate has set, you can store the berries between layers of parchment paper, in a closed container in the refrigerator.

PEANUT BUTTER DROPS

Five of these decadent peanut butter drops are the equivalent of 1/2 oz. of dark chocolate, and 1 2/3 tbsps. of peanut butter, so if you're a fool for peanut butter like I am, you can enjoy these every day of the week!

Yield: 28 peanut butter drops

Serving size: 5 drops

Ingredients:

- » One rounded ½ cup of cold, refrigerated, organic all natural peanut butter
- » ¼ cup of full fat, canned, organic coconut milk
- » 3 oz. of 72% cacao dark chocolate, chopped up or broken into small pieces

DIRECTIONS:

1. Line a baking sheet with parchment paper.
2. Place the chopped chocolate into a bowl.
3. Place the milk and oil into a sauce pan. Warm the milk mixture over a medium heat until it begins to bubble around the edges, but do not allow it to come to a boil.
4. Pour the heated milk mixture over the chocolate in the bowl and mix constantly, until all the chocolate has melted and is smooth.
5. Drop a teaspoon of peanut butter into the melted chocolate. Use a fork to swirl the chocolate around the peanut butter, and to remove the coated peanut butter drop from the bowl.
6. Place the chocolate coated drop onto the prepared baking sheet. When all the peanut butter drops are coated, place the baking sheet into the freezer for an hour or two to freeze.
7. When the drops are completely frozen, you can store them in layers, between parchment paper, in a covered container in the freezer. Take one or more out whenever you need a chocolate peanut butter fix!

COCONUT MILK ICE CREAM OR PUDDING

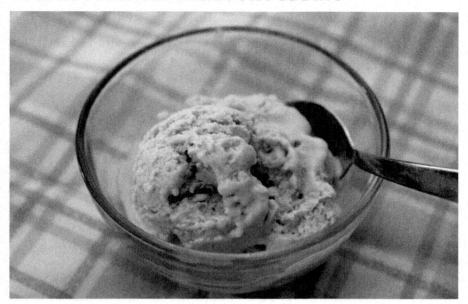

There are times when nothing but ice cream will do. Here's a creamy, thick, and delicious, non-dairy, version.

Yield: 2 cups

Serving size: ½ cup

Added sugar per serving: 1 tsp. – 1 ½ tsp.

Ingredients:

» 1 can (13.5 oz.) organic, full fat coconut milk

» 4 large, organic, pastured egg yolks

» 2 ½ tbsp. pure vanilla extract

» 1 ½-2 tbsp. organic raw honey

Directions:

1. Place the yolks into a small bowl and beat them with a wire whisk.

2. Place the coconut milk, and the vanilla into a small saucepan, on the stove top, over medium-low heat.

3. Heat the mixture stirring occasionally, until it is hot, but not boiling.

4. Add the honey to the pan, and stir.

5. While simultaneously whisking very quickly, pour a ladleful of the hot milk into the bowl of egg yolks. Repeat with two more ladleful's.

6. Now, add the yolks to the saucepan of milk and vanilla.

7. Whisking constantly, cook the ice cream mixture over medium-low heat. If you are cooking at the correct temperature, there should be a lot of steam around the edges of the pot, but no bubbles in the liquid.

8. Continue to cook the ice cream base for about 30 minutes, or until the ice cream base forms a custard that is similar in thickness to warm pudding.

9. Pour the custard into a glass dish, and cool on a wire rack for 40-50 minutes.

10. Mix the custard, and place the bowl into the refrigerator. Leave it in the refrigerator until it is completely chilled. It will continue to thicken as it chills. (If you like, you could stop here, and you would have a lovely vanilla pudding. Just cover the bowl, and store it in the refrigerator.)

11. Place the mixture into an ice cream maker and process. Cover the bowl and freeze. If you don't have an Ice cream maker, cover the bowl, and place it into the freezer. Stir the ice cream every 30 minutes, for 3-4 hours, or until it becomes ice cream. For ice cream pops, spoon the mixture into BPA free pop holders, and freeze until solid.

12. Enjoy! Store the leftovers covered, in the freezer. Once it has frozen solid, take the ice cream out of the freezer about 15-20 minutes before serving, for easier scooping. For easy removal of pops, run them under some warm water for a second or two.

FROZEN YOGURT POPS

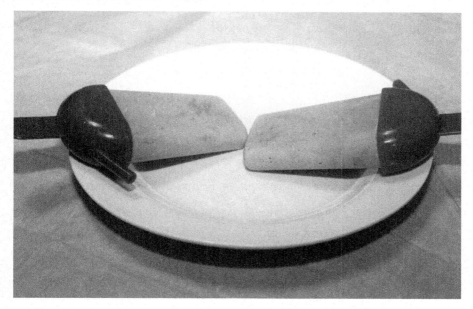

Okay, here's a way to get something healthy into your kids without them even knowing. This recipe is much healthier than the sugar laden frozen treats from the store. It's even a better alternative to juice pops, because even 100% juice has a lot of sugar, without a lot of fiber. Plus, your kids will have so much fun picking out the ingredients and helping to create this dessert (the combinations are almost limitless) & they'll be excitedly waiting for the pops to freeze!

Yield: 4 pops

Serving size: 1 pop

Added sugar per serving: ¾ tsp.

Ingredients:

- » 1 cup of fresh or frozen fruit of your choice
- » 1 cup of organic full fat, plain Greek yogurt
- » 2 tbsp. of homemade coconut milk (recipe in breakfast section)
- » 1 tbsp. organic raw honey

» 1 tbsp. stir-ins (coconut flakes, dark chocolate chips, chopped nuts, melted nut butter, etc.)

DIRECTIONS:

1. Place all the ingredients, except for the stir-ins, into a blender.
2. Blend until smooth.
3. Change the setting on your blender to whip, and whip until fluffy.
4. Add the stir-ins, and pulse to evenly disperse.
5. Pour into BPA free pop makers, and freeze for several hours.
6. Quick tip: For easy removal of pops, run them under some warm water for a second or two.

TIPS FOR DINING OUT & TRAVELING

For any plan to work it must be practical, and it must fit within the boundaries of everyday living. This includes traveling, eating out, and socializing. Here are a few tips to help you successfully navigate these normal everyday events.

BE PREPARED

If you know that you'll be traveling, pack some healthy snacks to take along with you. This will keep you from making a desperate choice during an inopportune moment of hunger. On a number of occasions, I have found myself on an unexpected road trip. I always grab a big bag of mixed nuts and some bottled water to take with me. I also keep tea bags in a plastic baggie, in my purse. Some other snacks ideas to take along when traveling would be: hard boiled eggs, apples, avocado, fresh vegetable strips, small containers of humus or nut butter, and dark chocolate. If you'll be on a long day trip, you can even pack breakfast and lunch to take with you, or you can plan ahead for what you will eat at rest stops.

FAST FOOD & DINERS

I've found that you can even make decent choices at fast food restaurants if you have to. For breakfast, there is nothing wrong with ordering a bacon and egg sandwich, or a sausage and egg sandwich, with a cup of coffee or tea. View the bun, roll, or flat bread, as nothing more than a holder for the filling. Eat the food between the bread, and toss the bread into the trash when you are done. Use heavy cream in your coffee or tea, or simply drink it black. For lunches, you can almost always order a salad with grilled chicken. If you can get to a diner, your options for meal choices on the road will broaden significantly. At a diner, you can order veggie omelets, large salads, beef, chicken, fish, and vegetables. Look for grilled, steamed, and baked, meats and vegetables. Avoid heavy sauces and tomato sauces which may contain flour, or added hidden sugars. Use olive oil and vinegar, or olive oil and fresh lemon juice for salad dressings. Try to pick foods which are prepared in a way that is similar, to how you would make them at home.

RESTAURANTS

If you can, go online and check the menu of the restaurant you're planning to visit ahead of time. This way you can make sure they have things on their menu that you want to eat, and you can even plan your meal before you get to the restaurant. There are lots of great meals to be had in almost any kind of restaurant without going off plan, and many restaurants are happy to make substitutions upon request. Lamb, shell fish, fish fillets, or a nice steak, are all good choices for an entrée. Fresh salads, guacamole, and vegetables that are sautéed, steamed, or served fresh, make nice sides. Enjoy a nice glass of red wine with your meal and have a cup of coffee, or a cappuccino with no whipped cream for dessert. Here's some different examples of the kinds of meals you might order in different types of restaurants.

In a Greek restaurant:

» Appetizers: Eggplant dip served with fresh veggies instead of pita's, or an olive tray with cubes of cheese.

» Entrees: Roasted lamb shank, kebabs, or a gyro platter with no pitas.

» Sides: Greek salad. Grilled or sautéed vegetables.

In a steak house:

» Appetizers: Shrimp cocktail, or Lobster & avocado salad.

» Entrees: Surf and turf, or Pork chops.

» Sides: Sautéed mushroom caps. Sautéed fresh baby spinach.

In a Mexican Restaurant:

» Appetizers: Guacamole and fresh vegetables.

» Entrees: Fajitas, or a steak, shrimp, or chicken dish.

» Sides: Refried beans. Salad.

In an Italian restaurant:

» Appetizers: Cold antipasto, or mussels Fra diablo.

» Entrées: Chicken cooked with asparagus in white wine, butter and lemon juice, or chicken with spinach, mushrooms, and tomato chunks, cooked in wine and butter.

» Sides: Zucchini rounds with parmesan cheese. A salad.

FAMILY GATHERINGS OR DINNER IN A FRIEND'S HOME.

Eating at someone else's home can be challenging especially if they don't eat the same way that you do. Whenever I visit my parents for example, I always bring lunch or dinner with me. It makes an easier day for them, and I don't have to worry about what I will eat.

Another idea when eating in someone else's home, is to ask if you can bring a dish to share. Bringing a dish from home will ensure that there's something available for you to eat.

If you're close to the host/hostess, you could also just ask them what they will be serving, and talk to them about what kinds of food are compliant with the plan. Don't expect them to change the whole menu, but if it's someone that you're close with they'll usually try to be accommodating in some way.

If you don't know your host that well, eat a small meal before going to the party or pack a snack for the ride home, just in case. At the party, select foods that are as compatible as possible with the plan.

EPILOGUE

THE DEFINITION OF HEALTH is not just the absence of disease. True health is a state of complete physical, mental, and social well-being. One of my greatest wishes, is the wish for you to reach this pinnacle of true health.

You may believe that you don't have the time to do things like cooking, exercising, journaling, or meditating, but you can make it happen. You may believe that taking the time to do these things for yourself is self-indulgent or selfish, but I want you to know, deep within yourself, that taking care of yourself, and the needs of your body, mind, and spirit, is one of the most unselfish things that you can do.

Know that your family and friends love you, and need you. You can't be fully present in their lives, if you're not fully present in your own. By taking care of yourself, not only will you be setting a great example for your kids and your family, but you'll be ensuring that you are well enough to be there for them, and to fully enjoy the life you share together.

What could be more unselfish? Remember on a plane the flight attendant always instructs you to use your own oxygen mask before trying to help others. That's because you can't be of use to someone else, if you yourself are in distress.

So, although you may need to take a bit more time for your own selfcare than you're used to, taking that time is neither selfish, nor self-indulgent, don't ever feel guilty about it. Instead, know that by taking care of yourself, you are making a better life for those you love, and that by being healthy and vibrant you'll be much better equipped to take care of your responsibilities, to handle life's challenges, and to enjoy your time on this earth.

When you reach the pinnacle of true health that I've discussed, you will have done it on your own, and with the support of those who love you. More support is also available. The official Healthy Body Connection – Book community on Facebook, is designed to be a loving, safe, and supportive place for you, and other members to ask questions, share experiences, ideas, recipes, and words of encouragement. You are invited to join us in the discussion at https://www.facebook.com/groups/399359440411607/, I hope to see you there.

For more information, recipes, tips, and the latest research, visit my blog at http://healthybodyconnection.com/ . Register for free with your email address.

Best wishes and love,

Lee Bomzer

ABOUT THE AUTHOR

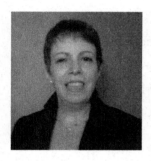 LEE BOMZER is a certified: Lifestyle Weight Management Specialist, Fitness Nutrition Coach, Personal Fitness Trainer, Group Fitness Instructor, Physique & Figure Training Specialist, and a member of the National Exercise & Sports Trainers Association. As an author and speaker, Lee continues to pursue her progressive education in the fields of nutrition, biology, endocrinology, psychology, and functional medicine.

For more information please visit http://healthybodyconnection.com

ACKNOWLEDGEMENTS

I WOULD LIKE TO THANK Dr. Rina Meyer for writing the forward to this book. You are one of the most beautiful people I have ever encountered. I am so amazed by you, and proud of you every day.

I would also like to thank Mr. Justin Sachs of Motivational Press, for seeing the potential in my work and for publishing this book.

To my brother, David. It seems like we are always headed down the path of life together, even when distance has separated us. Thank you so much for believing in me, and for encouraging me to keep striving for more. You were the catalyst for so many of my recent accomplishments, and I am grateful to have you as my brother.

To my daughter, Rachel. Thank you for everything that you do. You have been there assisting me, right from the start. I am very lucky to have such a generous and talented woman for a daughter.

Most importantly, I want to thank my husband and soul mate, Allan. You are my best friend, my strength, my hero, and so much more. We can do anything together, and I could have done none of this without you. Thank you for all the help you've given me, for loving me, and for always being so selflessly supportive of me. I am so incredibly blessed to have you for my husband.

RESOURCES

COMFORTABLE SUFFERING

Chatterjee, R How to make diseases disappear. TEDx Talks; You Tube (Dec 5, 2016) https://www.youtube.com/watch?v=gaY4m00wXp-w&t=6s&list=PLF8pwIT0dxjvks87hE46hb1rvwpKJ4a1M&index=2

THE PROBLEM

American Diabetes Association "Statistics About Diabetes" (12 December 2016) http://www.diabetes.org/diabetes-basics/statistics/?referrer=https://www.google.com/

Jeffrey S Bland, The Disease Delusion (HarperCollins, 2014) p. 6

Centers for Disease Control and Prevention "Childhood Obesity Facts" (27 August 2015) https://www.cdc.gov/healthyschools/obesity/facts.htm

Centers for Disease Control and Prevention "Heart Disease Facts" (10 August 2015) https://www.cdc.gov/heartdisease/facts.htm

Crane P, Walker R, Hubbard RA, Li G, Nathan DM, Zheng H, Haneuse S, Craft S, Montine TJ, Kahn SE, McCormick W, McCurry SM, Bowen JD, Larson EB, "Glucose Levels and Risk of Dementia" The New England Journal of Medicine. (26 September 2013) Vol. 369, p. 540-548

DiNicolantonio JJ, O'Keefe JH, Lucan SC "Added Fructose a Principal Driver of Type 2 Diabetes Mellitus and Its Consequences" Mayo Clinic Proceedings. (March 2015) Vol. 90, Issue 3, P. 372-381

Dufault R, Lukiw WJ, Crider R, Schnoll R, Wallinga D, Deth R "A macroepigenetic approach to identify factors responsible for the autism epidemic in the United States" Clinical Epigenetics. (10 April 2012) Vol. 4, Issue 6, DOI: 10.1186/1868-7083-4-6

Kushi, L. H., Doyle, C., McCullough, M., Rock, C. L., Demark-Wahnefried, W., Bandera, E. V., Gapstur, S., Patel, A. V., Andrews, K., Gansler, T. and The American Cancer Society 2010 Nutrition and Physical Activity Guidelines Advisory Committee (2012), "American Cancer Society guidelines on nutrition and physical activity for cancer prevention. CA: A Cancer Journal for Clinicians", The American Cancer Society Vol. 62, p.30-67, doi:10.3322/caac.20140

NIH National Heart, Lung, and Blood, Institute "What Are the Health Risks of Overweight and Obesity?" (13 July 2012). https://www.nhlbi.nih.gov/health/health-topics/topics/obe/risks

Ogden CL, Carroll MD, Kit BK, Flegal KM. "Prevalence of Childhood and Adult Obesity in the United States, 2011-2012." JAMA. (2014) Vol. 311, Issue 8, p.806-814. doi:10.1001/jama.2014.73

Andrew Stokes, Samuel H. Preston, "Deaths Attributable to Diabetes in the United States: Comparison of Data Sources and Estimation Approaches" PLoS ONE (25 January 2017) Vol 12, Issue 1, doi: 10.1371/journal.pone.0170219

The Lancet Diabetes & Endocrinology, "Cardiovascular disease, chronic kidney disease, and diabetes mortality burden of cardiometabolic risk factors from 1980 to 2010: a comparative risk assessment" (16 May 2014) Volume 2, Issue 8, p. 634-647

The Lancet, "Worldwide trends in diabetes since 1980: a pooled analysis of 751 population-based studies with 4·4 million participants" (06 April 2016) Vol. 387, Issue 10027, p. 1513-1530

Steven, Tokar, "Over Half of Alzheimer's Cases May Be Preventable, Say Researchers" University of California, San Francisco (19 July 2011) https//www.ucsf.edu/node/96545

Wisse, Brent E., "The inflammatory Syndrome: The Role of Adipose Tissue Cytokines in Metabolic Disorders Linked to Obesity" Journal of the American Society of Nephrology (1 November 2004) Vol. 15, no. 11, p. 2792-2800

World Health Organization "Obesity and overweight". (January 2015) http://www.who.int/mediacentre/factsheets/fs311/en/

THE FACTS

National Health Council "About Chronic Diseases". (29 July 2014) http://www.nationalhealthcouncil.org/sites/default/files/NHC_Files/Pdf_Files/AboutChronicDisease.pdf

The Lancet Diabetes & Endocrinology, "Cardiovascular disease, chronic kidney disease, and diabetes mortality burden of cardiometabolic risk factors from 1980 to 2010: a comparative risk assessment" (16 May 2014) Volume 2, Issue 8, p. 634-647

The Lancet, "Worldwide trends in diabetes since 1980: a pooled analysis of 751 population-based studies with 4·4 million participants" (6 April 2016) Volume 387, Issue 10027, p.1513-1530

Ram Weiss, Andrew A Bremer, and Robert H Lustig, "What is metabolic syndrome, and why are children getting it?" Annals of the New York Academy of Sciences. (2013) Vol. 1281, Issue 1, P. 123-140, doi:10.1111/nyas.12030.

World Health Organization "Diabetes Fact sheet" (March 2016) http://www.who.int/mediacentre/factsheets/fs312/en/

THE FIRST LAW, THE FIRST PROBLEM

Dominik D. Alexander, Paige E. Miller, Mary E. Van Elswyk, Connye N. Kuratko, Lauren C. Bylsma, "A Meta-Analysis of Randomized Controlled Trials and Prospective Cohort Studies of Eicosapentaenoic and Docosahexaenoic Long-Chain Omega-3 Fatty Acids and Coronary Heart Disease Risk" Mayo Clinic Proceedings (January 2017) Vol. 92, Issue 1,

p. 15-29

American Cancer Society "Make Exercise Work for You" (30 June 2014) (http://www.cancer.org/healthy/eathealthygetactive/getactive/make-exercise-work-for-you

American College of Gastroenterology Patient Education & Resource Center "Non-alcoholic Fatty Liver Disease (NAFLD)" (2012) http://patients.gi.org/topics/fatty-liver-disease-nafld/

American Heart Association "The American Heart Association's Diet and Lifestyle Recommendations" (24 October 2016)

American Institute for Cancer Research "AICR'S FOODS THAT FIGHT CANCER" (2016) http://www.aicr.org/foods-that-fight-cancer/?referrer=http://preventcancer.aicr.org/site/PageServer?pagename=foodsthatfightcancer_home

American Liver Foundation "Alcohol-Related Liver Disease" (14 January 2015) http://www.liverfoundation.org/abouttheliver/info/nafld/

Arizona Center for Integrative Medicine- University of Arizona "Phytochemicals and Your Health" (September 2010) https://integrativemedicine.arizona.edu/resources.html

Beth Ardoin, M.Ed., "Nutrition in preventative Medicine – Section 1, Proteins" (2004) http://www.uth.tmc.edu/courses/nutrition-module/section1/protein.html

Shane Bilsborough, Neil Mann, "A Review of Issues of Dietary Protein Intake in Humans" International Journal of Sport Nutrition and Exercise Metabolism (2006) Vol. 16, Issue 2, p. 129-152

BreastCancer.Org "Foods Containing Phytochemicals" (8 May 2013) http://www.breastcancer.org/tips/nutrition/reduce_risk/foods/phytochem

Cancer Treatment Centers of America "Super Foods for Fighting and Preventing Cancer" (2016) http://www.cancercenter.com/press-center/press-releases/2006/06/super-foods-for-fighting-and-preventing-cancer/

Emily Carey, Anna Wieckowska, William D. Carey, "Nonalcoholic Fatty Liver Disease" Cleveland Clinic (March 2013) http://www.cleve-landclinicmeded.com/medicalpubs/diseasemanagement/hepatology/nonalcoholic-fatty-liver-disease/

Donna Cataldo, Matthew Blair, "Protein Intake for Optimal Muscle Maintenance" American College of Sports Medicine (2015) https://www.acsm.org/docs/default-source/brochures/protein-intake-for-optimal-muscle-maintenance.pdf

Chia-Yu Chang, Der-Shin Ke, Jen-Yin Chen, "Essential Fatty Acids and Human Brain" Acta Neurologica Taiwanica (December 2009) Vol. 18, p. 231-241

Deepak Chopra, M.D, Rudy Tanzi, Ph.D., Super Genes (Harmony Books 2015) p.128-129

Cleveland Clinic "Heart Health Benefits of Chocolate" (2016) http://my.clevelandclinic.org/health/articles/benefits-of-chocolate-heart-health

Paul K. Crane, Rod Walker, Rebecca A. Hubbard, Ge Li, David M. Nathan, Hui Zheng, Sebastien Haneuse, Suzanne Craft, Thomas J. Montine, Steven E. Kahn, Wayne McCormick, Susan M. McCurry, James D. Bowen, Eric B. Larson, "Glucose Levels and Risk of Dementia" The New England Journal of Medicine (8 August 2013) Vol. 369, p.540-548

DiNicolantonio, O'Keefe, Lucan "Added Fructose" Mayo Clinic, p. 372-381

Endocrine Society "Testosterone decreases after ingestion of sugar (glucose)"(2017) https://www.endocrine.org/news-room/press-release archives/2010/testosteronedecreasesafteringestionofsugar

Phillip S. Ge, Bruce A. Runyon, "Treatment of Patients with Cirrhosis" The New England Journal of Medicine (25 August 2016) Vol.375, p. 767-777

Lee S. Gross, Li Li, Earl S. Ford, Simin Liu, "Increased consumption of refined carbohydrates and the epidemic of type 2 diabetes in the United States: an ecologic assessment 1-3" The American Journal of Clinical Nutrition (2004) Vol. 79, p. 774-779

Hallberg S Reversing Type 2 diabetes starts with ignoring the guidelines. TEDx Talks; You Tube (May 4, 2015) https://www.youtube.com/watch?v=da1vvigy5tQ

Harvard Health Publications – Harvard Medical School "Abundance of fructose not good for the liver, heart" (September 2011)

http://www.health.harvard.edu/heart-health/abundance-of-fructose-not-good-for-the-liver-heart

Harvard Health Publications – Harvard Medical School "Harvard Women's Health Watch, Foods that fight inflammation" (26 October 2015)

http://www.health.harvard.edu/staying-healthy/foods-that-fight-inflammation

Mark Hyman, MD, Eat Fat, Get Thin (Little, Brown and Company Hachette Book Group, 2016) p. 34

Caryn Jenky, "Protein Requirements for Athletes" Rice University (2016) http://www.rice.edu/~jenky/caryn/protein.html

Johns Hopkins Medicine Pathology "What causes pancreatic cancer?" (2016) http://pathology.jhu.edu/pc/BasicCauses.php?area=ba

M. D. Klok, S. Jakobsdottir, M. L. Drent, "The role of leptin and ghrelin in the regulation of food intake and body weight in humans: a review" Wiley Online Library (24 August 2006) http://onlinelibrary.wiley.com/doi/10.1111/j.1467-789X.2006.00270.x/full

Susanna C Larsson, Leif Bergkvist, Alicja Wolk, "Consumption of sugar and sugar-sweetened foods and the risk of pancreatic cancer in a prospective study1,2,3" The American Journal of Clinical Nutrition (2006) Vol. 84, No. 5, p.1171-1176

Belinda S Lennerz, David C Alsop, Laura M Holsen, Emily Stern, Rafael Rojas, Cara B Ebbeling, Jill M Goldstein, David S Ludwig, "Effects of dietary glycemic index on brain regions related to reward and craving in men" The American Journal of Clinical Nutrition (2013)

Vol. 98, No. 3, p. 641-647

Lobo V, Patil A, Phatak A, Chandra N. "Free radicals, antioxidants and functional foods: Impact on human health" Phcog Rev (2010) Vol. 4, p.118-126

David Ludwig M.D, PhD (11 May 2016) "Diabetes is by definition a state of carbohydrate intolerance, where the excess builds up as sugar in the blood. The pharmaceutical industry has devised creative ways to deal with this problem, including various types of insulin and drugs that make the body more sensitive to insulin. SGLT inhibitors are a pricey new category of drug that makes the kidneys excrete excess glucose (though with concerning side effects like urinary tract infections and greater risk for diabetic ketoacidosis). How about eating less processed carbohydrate? Then we wouldn't need to convert the kidneys into sugar disposal units." https://www.facebook.com/davidludwigmd/photos/a.1223378654344850.1073741828.1102248716457845/1349017305114317/?type=3&theater [Facebook update]. Retrieved from https://www.facebook.com/pg/davidludwigmd/posts/?ref=page_internal

David Ludwig, MD, Ph.D., Always Hungry (Hatchett Book Group, 2016) p. 6, 10-11, 56-57

Lustig R, M.D., FAT Chance (Hudson Street Press, 2013), p. 13, 34-35

Lustig R, Sugar: The Bitter Truth. University of California Television (UCTV); You Tube (Jul 30, 2009) https://www.youtube.com/watch?v=dBnniua6-oM

Anssi H. Manninen, "Metabolic Effects of the Very-Low-Carbohydrate Diets: Misunderstood "Villains" of Human Metabolism" Journal of the International Society of Sports Nutrition (December 2004) Vol. 2, p. 7-11

Dominique S. Michaud, Simin Liu, Edward Giovannucci, Walter C.

Willett, Graham A. Colditz, Charles S. Fuchs; "Dietary Sugar, Glycemic Load, and Pancreatic Cancer Risk in a Prospective Study." JNCI J Natl Cancer Inst (4 September 2002) Vol.94, Issue17, p. 1293-1300. doi: 10.1093/jnci/94.17.1293

Cornelia C. Metges, Christian A. Barth, "Metabolic Consequences of a High Dietary Protein Intake in Adulthood: Assessment of the Available Evidence" The Journal of Nutrition (1 April 2000) Vol. 130, No. 4, P. 886-889

NIH National Institute of Diabetes and Digestive and Kidney Diseases "Diagnosis of Diabetes and Prediabetes" (June 2014) https://sp-web.niddk.nih.gov/health-information/health-topics/Diabetes/diagnosis-diabetes-prediabetes/Pages/index.aspx

NIH National Institute of Diabetes and Digestive and Kidney Diseases "Nonalcoholic Steatohepatitis" (May 2014) https://www.niddk.nih.gov/health-information/liver-disease/nafld-nash/all-content

Official Website of Harvard Athletes "Recommended Daily Protein Intake – Female Athletes" (2014) http://www.gocrimson.com/information/strength_conditioning/nutrition/female_protein_intake

Official Website of Harvard Athletes "Recommended Daily Protein Intake – Male Athletes" (2014) http://www.gocrimson.com/information/strength_conditioning/nutrition/male_protein_intake

Physicians Committee for Responsible Medicine, "The Protein Myth" (2016) http://www.pcrm.org/health/diets/vsk/vegetarian-starter-kit-protein

M.J. Reed, R.W. Cheng, M. Simmonds, W. Richmond, V.H.T. James; "Dietary Lipids: an Additional Regulator of Plasma Levels of Sex Hormone Binding Globulin." The Journal of Clinical Endocrinology and Metabolism (2016) Vol. 64, Issue 5, p. 1083-1085 doi: 10.1210/jcem-64-5-1083

Melissa A. Schilling, "Unraveling Alzheimer's: Making Sense of the Relationship between Diabetes and Alzheimer's Disease" Journal of Alzheimer's Disease (January 2016) Vol. 51, p.961-977

Artemis Simopoulos, "The Importance of the Omega-6/Omega-3 Fatty Acid Ratio in Cardiovascular Disease and Other Chronic Diseases" Experimental Biology and Medicine (1 June 2008) Vol 233, Issue 6, p. 674-688

Gary Taubes, Why We Get Fat (First Anchor Books, 2011). p. 9-11

Nicole M Templeman, Sos Skovso, Melissa M Page, Gareth E Lim, and James D Johnson, "A causal role for hyperinsulinemia in obesity" Journal of Endocrinology (1 March 2017) Vol. 232, No. 3, p. R173-R183

The Lancet, "Worldwide trends in diabetes since 1980: a pooled analysis of 751 population-based studies with 4·4 million participants" (6 April 2016) Volume 387, Issue 10027, p. 1513-1530

Tokar, "Over Half" University of California, (19 July 2011) https//www.ucsf.edu/node/96545

Jeff S. Volek, William J. Kraemer, Jill A. Bush, Thomas Incledon, Mark Boetes, "Testosterone and cortisol in relationship to dietary nutrients and resistance exercise" Journal of Applied Physiology (Jan 1997) Vol. 82, Issue 1, p. 49-54

Eric C. Westman, "Is dietary carbohydrate essential for human nutrition?" The American Journal of Clinical Nutrition (May 2002) Vol. 75, Issue. 5, p. 951-953

Brent E. Wisse, "The Inflammatory Syndrome: The Role of Adipose Tissue Cytokines in Metabolic Disorders Linked to Obesity" Journal of the American Society of Nephrology (01 November 2004) Vol. 15 Issue 11, p. 2792-2800 doi: 10.1097/01.ASN.0000141966.69934.21

Ji Zhao, Lilin Li, Malcolm A Leissring, "Insulin-degrading enzyme is exported via an unconventional protein secretion pathway" Molecular Neurodegeneration (January 2009) Vol.4, p.4, Bio Med Central

Scratch that Reverse It!

Sandra Aamodt, "Never Diet Again" The New York Times, New York Edition (8 May 2016) p. SR1

Benjamin Caballero, "A Nutrition Paradox — Underweight and Obesity in Developing Countries" The New England Journal of Medicine (14 April 2005) Vol. 352, p.1514-1516

Erin Fothergill, Juen Guo, Lilian Howard, Jennifer C. Kerns, Nicolas D. Knuth, Robert Brychta, Kong Y. Chen, Monica C. Skarulis, Mary Walter, Peter J. Walter, Kevin D. Hall, "Persistent metabolic adaptation 6 years after "The Biggest Loser" competition" Obesity (August 2016) Vol. 24, Issue 8, p. 1599–1821

Joel Fuhrman, "The Dangers of Weight Cycling (Yo – Yo Dieting)" Dr. Fuhrman Smart Nutrition. Superior Health. (2016) https://www.drfuhrman.com/learn/library/articles/79/the-dangers-of-weight-cycling-yo-yo-dieting

Gina Kolata "That Lost Weight? The Body Finds It." The New York Times, New York Edition (2 May 2016) p. A1

K H Pietiläinen, S E Saarni, J Kaprio, and A Rissanen "Does dieting make you fat? A twin study" International Journal of Obesity (2012) Vol. 36, P. 456-464

Gerard E. Mullin, M.D., The Gut Balance Revolution (Rodale Inc. 2014) p. 2-3

World Health Organization, "What is malnutrition- Online Q&A" (8 July 2016) http://www.who.int/features/qa/malnutrition/en/

Hormones, and Lifestyle

Estrogen and Testosterone

Joel S. Finkelstein, Hang Lee, Sherri-Ann M. Burnett-Bowie, J. Carl Pallais, Elaine W. Yu, Lawrence F. Borges, Brent F. Jones, Christopher V. Barry, Kendra E. Wulczyn, Bijoy J. Thomas, Benjamin Z. Leder, "Gonadal

Steroids and Body Composition, Strength, and Sexual Function in Men" The New England Journal of Medicine (12 September 2013) Vol. 369, No. 11, p. 999-1010

Hormone Health Network "FACT SHEET -Low Testosterone and Men's Health" (2017) http://www.hormone.org/questions-and-answers/2010/low-testosterone-and-mens-health

Hormone Health Network "What is Estrogen?" (2017) http://www.hormone.org/diseases-and-conditions/womens-health/what-is-estrogen

M. E. J. Lean, D. Malkova, "Altered gut and adipose tissue hormones in overweight and obese individuals: cause or consequence?" International Journal of Obesity (2016) Vol. 40, p. 622-632; doi:10.1038/ijo.2015.220

Christiane Northrup, "What Are the Symptoms of Estrogen Dominance?" Christiane Northrup, M.D. (2016) http://www.drnorthrup.com/estrogen-dominance/

Stress and Cortisol

Encyclopedia Britannica. Encyclopedia Britannica Online. "Cortisol" (17 May 2016) http://www.britannica.com/science/cortisol>.

Michael Randall "The Physiology of Stress: Cortisol and the Hypothalamic-Pituitary-Adrenal Axis" (3 February 2011) Dartmouth Undergraduate Journal of Sciences http://dujs.dartmouth.edu/2011/02/the-physiology-of-stress-cortisol-and-the-hypothalamic-pituitary-adrenal-axis/#.WJCqwFMrKM8

Getting your ZZZ's

Christian Benedict, Samantha J. Brooks, Owen G. O'Daly, Markus S. Almèn, Arvid Morell, Karin Öberg, Malin Gingnell, Bernd Schultes, Manfred Hallschmid, Jan-Erik Broman, Elna-Marie Larsson, Helgi B. Schiöth, "Acute Sleep Deprivation Enhances the Brain's Response to Hedonic Food Stimuli: An fMRI Study." The Journal of Clinical

Endocrinology and Metabolism (1 March 2012) Vol. 97, Issue 3, p. E443-E447. doi: 10.1210/jc.2011-2759

Andrew D. Calvin, Naima Covassin, Walter K. Kremers, Taro Adachi, Paula Macedo, Felipe N. Albuquerque, Jan Bukartyk, Diane E. Davison, James A. Levine, Prachi Singh, Shihan Wang, Virend K. Somers, "Experimental Sleep Restriction Causes Endothelial Dysfunction in Healthy Humans" Journal of the American Heart Association (25 November 2014) Vol. 3, e001143 doi.org/10.1161/JAHA.114.001143

Cedars-Sinai, "Endothelial Function Testing" (2016) https://www.cedars-sinai.edu/Patients/Programs-and-Services/Womens-Heart-Center/Services/Endothelial-Function-Testing.aspx

Michel Félétou, "The Endothelium, Part 1: Multiple Functions of the Endothelial Cells—Focus on Endothelium-Derived Vasoactive Mediators" NCBI Bookshelf (2011) https://www.ncbi.nlm.nih.gov/books/NBK57149/

Roo Killick, Siobhan Banks, Peter Y. Liu, "Implications of Sleep Restriction and Recovery on Metabolic Outcomes" The Journal of Clinical Endocrinology and Metabolism (1 November 2012) Vol. 97, Issue 11, p. 3876-3890. doi: 10.1210/jc.2012-1845

Tae Won Kim, Jong-Hyun Jeong, and Seung-Chul Hong, "The Impact of Sleep and Circadian Disturbance on Hormones and Metabolism," International Journal of Endocrinology, (24 February 2015) vol. 2015, ID 591729, p. 2015-2024. doi:10.1155/2015/591729

A. N. Vgontzas, E. Zoumakis, E. O. Bixler, H.-M. Lin, H. Follett, A. Kales, G. P. Chrousos, "Adverse Effects of Modest Sleep Restriction on Sleepiness, Performance, and Inflammatory Cytokines" The Journal of Clinical Endocrinology and Metabolism (01 May 2004) Vol. 89, Issue 5, p. 2119-2126. doi: 10.1210/jc.2003-031562

The Body in Motion/Use it or Lose it

James A. Levine, "Sick of sitting" Diabetologia (August 2015), Volume 58, Issue 8, pp 1751-1758

James A. Levine, "What are the risks of sitting too much?" Mayo Clinic (04 September 2015) http://www.mayoclinic.org/healthy-lifestyle/adult-health/expert-answers/sitting/faq-20058005

John Hopkins Medicine - Health Library "Risks of Physical Inactivity" (2016)_____http://www.hopkinsmedicine.org/healthlibrary/conditions/cardiovascular_diseases/risks_of_physical_inactivity_85,p00218/

World Health Organization - Media center "Physical inactivity a leading cause of disease and disability, warns WHO" (4 April 2002) http://www.who.int/mediacentre/news/releases/release23/en/

Toxins

Bland, The Disease Delusion (HarperCollins, 2014) p. 133

Jonathan G. Boucher, Shaimaa Ahmed, Ella Atlas "Bisphenol S Induces Adipogenesis in Primary Human Preadipocytes From Female Donors" Endocrinology (1 April 2016) Vol. 157, Issue 4, p. 1397-1407

Celiac Disease Foundation "CELIAC DISEASE SYMPTOMS" (12 March 2016) https://celiac.org/celiac-disease/understanding-celiac-disease-2/celiacdiseasesymptoms/

Celiac Disease Foundation "NON-CELIAC WHEAT SENSITIVITY" (2106) https://celiac.org/celiac-disease/understanding-celiac-disease-2/non-celiac-gluten-sensitivity-2/

Celiac Disease Foundation "SOURCES OF GLUTEN" (2016) https://celiac.org/live-gluten-free/glutenfreediet/sources-of-gluten/

Chopra, Tanzi, Super Genes (Harmony Books 2015) p.134

Sandro Drago, Ramzi El Asmar, Mariarosaria Di Pierro, Maria Grazia Clemente, Amit Tripathi Anna Sapone, Manjusha Thakar, Giuseppe Iacono, Antonio Carroccio, Cinzia D'Agate, Tarcisio Not, Lucia Zampini, Carlo

Catassi, and Alessio Fasano, "Gliadin, zonulin and gut permeability: Effects on celiac and non-celiac intestinal mucosa and intestinal cell lines" Scandinavian Journal of Gastroenterology (2006) Vol. 41, Issue 4, p. 408-419

Hollon, J.; Puppa, E.L.; Greenwald, B.; Goldberg, E.; Guerrerio, A.; Fasano, A., "Effect of Gliadin on Permeability of Intestinal Biopsy Explants from Celiac Disease Patients and Patients with Non-Celiac Gluten Sensitivity." Nutrients (27 February 2015), Vol. 7, p. 1565-1576.

Mayo Clinic Diseases and Conditions "Milk Allergy Symptoms" (07 August 2014) http://www.mayoclinic.org/diseases-conditions/milk-allergy/basics/symptoms/con-20032147

NIH U.S. National Library of Medicine – Genetics Home Reference "What is a cell?" (2016) https://ghr.nlm.nih.gov/primer/basics/cell

NIH U.S. National Library of Medicine – Genetics Home Reference "What is DNA?" (2016) https://ghr.nlm.nih.gov/primer/basics/dna

Karin de Punder, Leo Pruimboom, "The Dietary Intake of Wheat and other Cereal Grains and Their Role in Inflammation" Nutrients (2013) Vol. 5, p. 771-787

Melanie Uhde, Mary Ajamian, Giacomo Caio, Roberto De Giorgio, Alyssa Indart, Peter H Green, Elizabeth C Verna, Umberto Volta, Armin Alaedini, "Intestinal cell damage and systemic immune activation in individuals reporting sensitivity to wheat in the absence of coeliac disease" BMJ-Gut (2016) Vol. 65, p. 1930-1937. doi:10.1136/gutjnl-2016-311964

University of Colorado, Colorado Springs "Simple Elimination Diet" (2016) http://www.uccs.edu/Documents/healthcircle/pnc/health-topics/Allergy%20Elimination%20Diet.pdf

Ami R. Zota, Cassandra A. Phillips, Susanna D. Mitro, "Recent Fast Food Consumption and Bisphenol A and Phthalates Exposures among the U.S. Population in NHANES, 2003–2010" Environmental Health Perspectives (13 April 2016) Vol.124, p. 1521–1528 http://dx.doi.org/10.1289/ehp.1510803

The Microbiome

Bland, The Disease Delusion (Harper Collins, 2014) p.103, 234

Marla Vacek Broadfoot "Rise of the Microbiome" Discovery's Edge - Mayo Clinic's Research Magazine (February 2016) http://discoverysedge. mayo.edu/2016/01/08/rise-of-the-microbiome/

Kirsty Brown, Daniella DeCoffe, Erin Molcan, Deanna L. Gibson, "Diet-Induced Dysbiosis of the Intestinal Microbiota and the Effects on Immunity and Disease" Nutrients (21 August 2012) Vol. 4, Issue 8, p. 1095-1119; doi:10.3390/nu4081095

Jessica Stoller-Conrad, "Microbes Help Produce Serotonin in Gut" Caltech (04 September 2015) https://www.caltech.edu/news/microbes-help-produce-serotonin-gut-46495

Cornell University, Department of Microbiology "Low G+C Gram Positive Bacteria" (2016) https://micro.cornell.edu/research/epulopiscium/low-g-and-c-gram-positive-bacteria

Ludovic Giloteaux, Julia K. Goodrich, William A. Walters, Susan M. Levine, Ruth E. Ley, Maureen R. Hanson, "Reduced diversity and altered composition of the gut microbiome in individuals with myalgic encephalomyelitis/chronic fatigue syndrome" Microbiome (23 June 2016) Volume 4, Issue 30, DOI: 10.1186/s40168-016-0171-4

Hyman, MD, Eat Fat, Get Thin (Little, Brown and Company Hachette Book Group, 2016) p. 27

Dr. Frank Lipman, "Why Your Microbiome is Important to Your Health" The Be Well Blog (07 March 2016) https://www.bewell.com/blog/why-your-microbiome-is-important-to-your-health/

Moises Velasquez-Manoff, "Educate Your Immune System" The New York Times-New York edition (5 June 2016), p. SR1

James McIntosh, "Serotonin: Facts, What Does Serotonin Do?" Medical New Today (29 April 2016) http://www.medicalnewstoday.com/kc/serotonin-facts-232248

Mullin, M.D., The Gut Balance Revolution (Rodale Inc. 2014) p.6-7

Judy Palken, "Prebiotics: What, where, and how to get them" UMASS Center for Microbiome Research (13 April 2015) https://umasscmr. wordpress.com/2015/04/14/prebiotics-what-where-and-how-to-get-them/

Kenneth Todar, PhD, "Bacterial Endotoxin" Todar's Online Textbook of Bacteriology (2012) http://textbookofbacteriology.net/endotoxin.html

Marius Trøseid, Torunn K. Nestvold, Knut Rudi, Hanne Thoresen, Erik W. Nielsen, Knut T. Lappegård, "Plasma Lipopolysaccharide Is Closely Associated with Glycemic Control and Abdominal Obesity" Diabetes Care (Nov 2013) Vol 36, Issue 11, p. 3627-3632

University of Wisconsin Integrative Medicine, "Probiotics and Prebiotics: Frequently Asked Questions" (2016) http://www.fammed. wisc.edu/files/webfm-uploads/documents/outreach/im/handout_probiotics_patient.pdf

The Myth

Dietary Guidelines Advisory Committee, "History of Dietary Guidance Development in the United States and the Dietary Guidelines for Americans" (2017) https://health.gov/dietaryguidelines/2015-binder/meeting1/historycurrentuse.aspx

Eating Right PDF "Choose Your Low-Cholesterol Heart Healthy Diet" (1996) http://dbhmd.org/resources/Eating+Right.pdf

EUFIC "Food-based dietary guidelines in Europe" (01 October 2009) http://www.eufic.org/en/healthy-living/article/food-based-dietary-guidelines-in-europe

Pavel Grasgruber, Martin Sebera, Eduard Hrazdira, Sylva Hrebickova, Jan Cacek, "Food consumption and the actual statistics of cardiovascular diseases: an epidemiological comparison of 42 European countries." (27 September 2016) Food & Nutrition Research, Vol. 60, doi: http://dx.doi.

org/10.3402/fnr.v60.31694

David S. Ludwig, "Lifespan Weighed Down by Diet" JAMA. (7 June 2016) Vol. 315, No.21,

P. 2269-2270. doi:10.1001/jama.2016.3829

Nutrition and Your Health: Dietary Guidelines for Americans, 1990 [PDF – 478 KB], https://health.gov/dietaryguidelines/1990thin.pdf?_ga =1.153568955.202208470.1485978553

Office of Disease Prevention and Health Promotion, "Nutrition and Your Health: Dietary Guidelines for Americans, 1990 [PDF – 478 KB]" (2017) https://health.gov/dietaryguidelines/1990.asp

Office of Disease Prevention and Health Promotion, "Report of the Dietary Guidelines Advisory Committee on the Dietary Guidelines for Americans, 1985 [PDF – 1.1 MB]" (2017) https://health.gov/dietaryguidelines/1985.asp

Christopher E. Ramsden, Daisy Zamora, Sharon Majchrzak-Hong, Keturah R. Faurot, Steven K. Broste, Robert P. Frantz, John M. Davis, Amit Ringel, Chirayath M. Suchindran, Joseph R. Hibbeln, "Re-evaluation of the traditional diet-heart hypothesis: analysis of recovered data from Minnesota Coronary Experiment (1968-73)" BMJ (12 April 2016) 353: i1246

The Lancet Diabetes & Endocrinology, Volume 2, Issue 8, p. 634-647 "Cardiovascular disease, chronic kidney disease, and diabetes mortality burden of cardiometabolic risk factors from 1980 to 2010: a comparative risk assessment"

US Department of Human Health and Services, "History of Dietary Guidelines for Americans -Nutrition and Your Health: Dietary Guidelines for Americans, 1980" https://health.gov/dietaryguidelines/history.htm#6,

US Department of Human Health and Services, "History of Dietary Guidelines for Americans -Nutrition and Your Health: Dietary Guidelines for Americans, 1985" https://health.gov/dietaryguidelines/history.htm#5

US Department of Human Health and Services, "Nutrition and Your Health: Dietary Guidelines for Americans" (1980) https://health.gov/dietaryguidelines/1980thin.pdf?_ga=1.227435294.202208470.1485978553

US Department of Human Health and Services, "Nutrition and Your Health: Dietary Guidelines for Americans" (1985) https://health.gov/dietaryguidelines/1985thin.pdf?_ga=1.220163738.202208470.1485978553

Peter Whoriskey, "This study 40 years ago could have reshaped the American diet. But it was never fully published." The Washington Post (12 April 2016) https://www.washingtonpost.com/news/wonk/wp/2016/04/12/this-study-40-years-ago-could-have-reshaped-the-american-diet-but-it-was-never-fully-published/?utm_term=.71248273b55a

World Health Organization "Obesity and overweight". (January 2015) http://www.who.int/mediacentre/factsheets/fs311/en/

The Approach

Kelly M. Adams, W. Scott Butsch, and Martin Kohlmeier, "The State of Nutrition Education at US Medical Schools," Journal of Biomedical Education, (11 January 2015) vol. 2015, Article ID 357627, 7 pages. doi:10.1155/2015/357627

David Blackburn, Thomas W. Wilson, "Antihypertensive medications and blood sugar: Theories and implications" Canadian Journal of Cardiology (March 2006) Vol. 22, Issue 3, p. 229-233

Bland, "The Disease Delusion" (Harper Collins, 2014) p.13, 24-26, 86

Henna Cederberg, Alena Stančáková, Nagendra YaluriShalem, ModiJohanna Kuusisto, Markku Laakso, "Increased risk of diabetes with statin treatment is associated with impaired insulin sensitivity and insulin secretion: a 6 year follow-up study of the METSIM cohort" Diabetologia (May 2015), Vol. 58, Issue 5, p. 1109–1117

Chopra, Tanzi, "Super Genes" (Harmony Books 2015) p.1-5

Michael E. Delgado, Nasar U. Ahmed, "Physician-Delivered Dietary Counseling: A Review." Journal of Nature and Science (JNSCI), (2016) Vol. 2, No. 5, e192.

Harvard T.H. Chan School of Public Health, "Healthy lifestyle could prevent half of all cancer deaths" (2016) https://www.hsph.harvard.edu/news/hsph-in-the-news/healthy-lifestyle-could-prevent-half-of-all-cancer-deaths/

Mark Hyman, M.D., "The Biggest "Drug" to Reverse or Prevent Heart Disease Isn't a Medication" Dr. Hyman (21 April 2016) http://drhyman.com/blog/2016/04/21/the-biggest-drug-to-reverse-or-prevent-heart-disease-isnt-a-medication

David Ludwig M.D, PhD (11 May 2016) "Diabetes is by definition a state of carbohydrate intolerance, where the excess builds up as sugar in the blood. The pharmaceutical industry has devised creative ways to deal with this problem, including various types of insulin and drugs that make the body more sensitive to insulin. SGLT inhibitors are a pricey new category of drug that makes the kidneys excrete excess glucose (though with concerning side effects like urinary tract infections and greater risk for diabetic ketoacidosis). How about eating less processed carbohydrate? Then we wouldn't need to convert the kidneys into sugar disposal units." https://www.facebook.com/davidludwigmd/photos/a.1223378654344850.1073741828.1102248716457845/1349017305114317/?type=3&theater [Facebook update]. Retrieved from https://www.facebook.com/pg/davidludwigmd/posts/?ref=page_internal

Mukherjee S. Soon We'll Cure Diseases with a Cell, Not a Pill TED Talks; You Tube (October 28, 2015) https://www.youtube.com/watch?v=qG_YmIPFO68&t=8s

NIH National Institute of Diabetes and Digestive and Kidney Diseases "Diagnosis of Diabetes and Prediabetes" (June 2014) https://sp-web.niddk.nih.gov/health-information/health-topics/Diabetes/diagnosis-diabetes-prediabetes/Pages/index.aspx

NYU Langone Medical Center, "Study Finds Physicians Want to Learn More About Diet & Cardiovascular Disease Prevention" (16 March 2015) http://nyulangone.org/press-releases/study-finds-physicians-want-to-learn-more-about-diet-cardiovascular-disease-prevention

Charles Ornstein, Ryann Grochowski Jones, and Mike Tigas, "Now There's Proof: Docs Who Get Company Cash Tend to Prescribe More Brand-Name Meds" ProPublica, (March 17, 2016) https://www.propublica.org/article/doctors-who-take-company-cash-tend-to-prescribe-more-brand-name-drugs#republish

Pfizer, "ARICEPT U.S. Patient Product Information (PDF)" http://www.pfizer.com/products/product-detail/aricept

QuintilesIMS Institute, "IMS Health Study: U.S. Drug Spending Growth Reaches 8.5 Percent in 2015" (14 Apr 2016) http://www.imshealth.com/en/thought-leadership/quintilesims-institute/news-and-press/ims-health-study-us-drug-spending-growth-reaches-8.5-percent-in-2015

Mingyang Song, Edward Giovannucci, "Preventable Incidence and Mortality of Carcinoma Associated with Lifestyle Factors Among White Adults in the United States" JAMA Oncol. (1 July 2016) Vol.2, No. 9, p.1154-1161. doi:10.1001/jamaoncol.2016.0843

Victoza, "Selected Important Safety Information" (2017) https://www.victozapro.com/safety-and-tolerability.html

Organic, Wild, and Pasture Raised Foods

Kate Clancy, "Greener Pastures" Union of Concerned Scientists (March 2006) http://www.ucsusa.org/food_and_agriculture/solutions/advance-sustainable-agriculture/greener-pastures.html#.WJOSoVMrKM8

Cynthia A Daley, Amber Abbott, Patrick S Doyle, Glenn A Nader, Stephanie Larson, "A review of fatty acid profiles and antioxidant content in grass-fed and grain-fed beef" (10 March 2010) Nutrition Journal Vol. 9, Issue 10, DOI: 10.1186/1475-2891-9-10

Jillian P. Frya, David C. Lovea, Graham K. MacDonaldd, Paul C. Weste, Peder M. Engstrome, Keeve E. Nachmana, Robert S. Lawrencea, "Environmental health impacts of feeding crops to farmed fish" Environment International (May 2016) Vol. 91, p.201-214

Nicole Greenfield, "The Smart Seafood Buying Guide" Natural Resource Defense Council (26 August 2015) https://www.nrdc.org/stories/smart-seafood-buying-guide

Jo Robinson "Health Benefits of Grass-Fed Products" Eat Wild (2016) http://www.eatwild.com/healthbenefits.htm

D C Rule, K S Broughton, S M Shellito, G Maiorano "Comparison of muscle fatty acid profiles and cholesterol concentrations of bison, beef cattle, elk, and chicken." (2002) Journal of animal science Vol. 80, No. 5, p.1202-1211. doi:10.2527/2002.8051202x

Washington State Department of Health, "Health Fish Guide" (2016) http://www.doh.wa.gov/CommunityandEnvironment/Food/Fish/HealthyFishGuide

A Rainbow of Fruits and Vegetables

Healthy Balance Nutrition LLC "Eating the Rainbow: From the Institute for Functional Medicine, Phytonutrient-Spectrum-Comprehensive Guide.pdf. Phytonutrient-Spectrum-Comprehensive-Guide" (2014) http://healthybalancenutritionllc.com/resources/

The University of Arizona – Arizona center for Integrative Medicine, "Phytochemicals and Your Health" (2010) https://integrativemedicine.arizona.edu/resources.html

Fresh Herbs and Spices

Winston J Craig, "Health-promoting properties of common herbs" The American Journal of Clinical Nutrition (September 1999) Vol.70, no. 3, p. 491s-499s

Joanna Hlebowicz, Gassan Darwiche, Ola Björgell, Lars-Olof Almér, "Effect of cinnamon on postprandial blood glucose, gastric emptying, and satiety in healthy subjects" The American Journal of Clinical Nutrition (June 2007) Vol. 85, No. 6, P. 1552-1556

Christine M. Kaefer, John A. Milne," The role of herbs and spices in cancer prevention" Journal of Nutritional Biochemistry (June 2008) Volume 19, Issue 6, p.347-361

Subodh Kumar, Kiran Saxena, Uday N. Singh, Ravi Saxena, "Anti-inflammatory action of ginger: A critical review in anemia of inflammation and its future aspects" International Journal of Herbal Medicine (14 October 2013) Vol. 1, Issue 4, p.16-20, ISSN 2321-2187

Steven Masley, MD, Mindbodygreen "9 Spices & Herbs Everyone Should Eat For Optimal Health: A Doctor Explains"(18 January 2016) http://www.mindbodygreen.com/0-23253/9-spices-herbs-everyone-should-eat-for-optimal-health-a-doctor-explains.html

Michigan Medicine University of Michigan, "Cooking with Herbs and Spices" (May 2013) https://www.med.umich.edu/.../cookingwithherbsandspices-0513.pdf

Michigan Medicine University of Michigan, "Healing Foods Pyramid" (2017) www.med.umich.edu/umim/food-pyramid/seasonings.html

Sahdeo Prasad, Amit K. Tyagi, "Ginger and Its Constituents: Role in Prevention and Treatment of Gastrointestinal Cancer" Gastroenterology Research and Practice, (2015) Vol. 2015, Article ID 142979, 11 pages. doi:10.1155/2015/142979

Full Fat Dairy Products

Jiansong Bao, Fiona Atkinson, Peter Petocz, Walter C Willett, Jennie C Brand-Miller, "Prediction of postprandial glycemia and insulinemia in lean, young, healthy adults: glycemic load compared with carbohydrate content alone" The American Journal of Clinical Nutrition (May 2011) Vol. 93, No. 5, p.984-996

C Hoppe, C Mølgaard, C Dalum, A Vaag, K F Michaelsen, "Differential effects of casein versus whey on fasting plasma levels of insulin, IGF-1 and IGF-1/IGFBP-3: results from a randomized 7-day supplementation study in prepubertal boys" European Journal of Clinical Nutrition (2009) Vol. 63, p.1076–1083; doi:10.1038/ejcn.2009.34

Mikael Nilsson, Marianne Stenberg, Anders H Frid, Jens J Holst, Inger ME Björck, "Glycemia and insulinemia in healthy subjects after lactose-equivalent meals of milk and other food proteins: the role of plasma amino acids and incretins" The American Journal of Clinical Nutrition (November 2004) Vol. 80, No. 5, p. 1246-1253

Larry A. Tucker, Andrea Erickson, James D. LeCheminant, Bruce W. Bailey, "Dairy Consumption and Insulin Resistance: The Role of Body Fat, Physical Activity, and Energy Intake" Journal of Diabetes Research (2015) Vol.2015, Article ID 206959, 11 pages, doi:10.1155/2015/206959

Whole Eggs

Grasgruber, Sebera, Hrazdira, Hrebickova, Cacek, "Food consumption and the actual statistics of cardiovascular diseases" (27 September 2016) Food & Nutrition Research, Vol 60, P. 31694. doi: 10.3402/fnr.v60.31694

Jane Higdon, Victoria J. Drake, Barbara Delage, "Choline" Oregon State University – Linus Pauling Institute (2015) http://lpi.oregonstate.edu/mic/other-nutrients/choline

Jon White, Daniel I. Swerdlow, David Preiss, Zammy Fairhurst-Hunter, Brendan J. Keating, Folkert W. Asselbergs, Naveed Sattar, MD, Steve E.

Humphries, Aroon D. Hingorani, Michael V. Holmes, "Association of Lipid Fractions with Risks for Coronary Artery Disease and Diabetes." (September 2016) JAMA Cardiol. Vol. 1, No.6, p.692-699. doi:10.1001/jamacardio.2016.1884

Steven H Zeisel, Kerry-Ann da Costa; "Choline: an essential nutrient for public health." Nutrition Reviews (2014) Vol. 67, Issue 11, p. 615-623. doi: 10.1111/j.1753-4887.2009.00246.x

Healthy Fats and Omega 3's

Alexander, Miller, Van Elswyk, Kuratko, Bylsma, "A Meta-Analysis of Randomized Controlled Trials and Prospective Cohort Studies of Eicosapentaenoic and Docosahexaenoic Long-Chain Omega-3 Fatty Acids and Coronary Heart Disease Risk" Mayo Clinic Proceedings (January 2017) Vol. 92, Issue 1, p. 15-29

Simopoulos, "The Importance of the Omega-6/Omega-3 Fatty Acid Ratio in Cardiovascular Disease and Other Chronic Diseases" Experimental Biology and Medicine (1 June 2008) Vol 233, Issue 6, p. 674-688.

Dark Chocolate

Diederik Esser, Monica Mars, Els Oosterink, Angelique Stalmach, Michael Müller, Lydia A. Afman, "Dark chocolate consumption improves leukocyte adhesion factors and vascular function in overweight men" The FASEB Journal, (March 2014) Vol. 28, No. 3, p.1464-1473.

Davide Grassi, Stefano Necozione, Cristina Lippi, Giuseppe Croce, Letizia Valeri, Paolo Pasqualetti, Giovambattista Desideri, Jeffrey B. Blumberg, Claudio Ferri, "Cocoa Reduces Blood Pressure and Insulin Resistance and Improves Endothelium-Dependent Vasodilation in

Hypertensives" <u>Hypertension</u>. (28 July 2005) Vol. 46, p.398-405. doi: 10.1161/01.HYP.0000174990.46027.70

Franz H. Messerli, "Chocolate Consumption, Cognitive Function, and Nobel Laureates" <u>The New England Journal of Medicine</u> (18 October 2012) Vol. 367, p.1562-1564. DOI: 10.1056/NEJMon1211064

Ivan M. Petyaev, Pavel Y. Dovgalevsky, Natalia E. Chalyk, Victor Klochkov, Nigel H. Kyl, "Reduction in blood pressure and serum lipids by lycosome formulation of dark chocolate and lycopene in prehypertension." (17 September 2014) <u>Food and Science Nutrition</u>, Vol. 2, p. 744–750. doi:10.1002/fsn3.169

Water

About Anne Marie Helmenstine, "Question: How Much of Your Body Is Water? "<u>About Education</u> (31 October 2016) http://chemistry.about.com/cs/foodchemistry/a/aa070803a.htm

Julia McHugh, Nancy R. Keller, Martin Appalsamy, Steven A. Thomas, Satish R. Raj, André Diedrich, Italo Biaggioni, Jens Jordan, David Robertson, "Portal Osmopressor Mechanism Linked to Transient Receptor Potential Vanilloid 4 and Blood Pressure Control" (May 19, 2010) <u>Hypertension Vol.55, p.1438-1443. doi:</u> 10.1161/HYPERTENSIONAHA.110.151860

David H. Nguyen "What Critical Role Does Water Play in Homeostasis?" <u>Seattlepi</u> (2017) <u>http://education.seattlepi.com/critical-role-water-play-homeostasis-4708.html</u>

Randall K. Packer, "How long can the average person survive without water?" Scientific American (9 December 2002) <u>https://www.scientificamerican.com/article/how-long-can-the-average/</u>

Coffee & Tea

US Food & Drug Administration, "Medicines in my Home: Caffeine and Your Body" (2007) http://www.fda.gov/downloads/UCM200805.pdf

American Institute for Cancer Research, "AICR'S Foods that Fight Cancer, Coffee" (2016) http://www.aicr.org/foods-that-fight-cancer/coffee.html

Shilpa N. BhupathirajuAn, PanJoAnn E. Manson, Walter C. Willett, Rob M. Van Dam, Frank B. Hu, "Changes in coffee intake and subsequent risk of type 2 diabetes: three large cohorts of US men and women" Diabetologia (July 2014) Volume 57, Issue 7, pp 1346-1354

Silvio Buscemi, Stefano Marventano, Mariagrazia Antoci, Antonella Cagnetti, Gabriele Castorina, Fabio Galvano, Marina Marranzano, Antonio Mistretta, "Coffee and metabolic impairment: An updated review of epidemiological studies" NFS Journal (February 2016) Volume 3, August 2016, P. 1-7. doi: 10.1016/j.nfs.2016.02.001

Karrie Heneman, Sheri Zidenberg-Cherr, "Some Facts About Catechins" (November 2007) UC Cooperative Extension Center for Health and Nutrition Research Department of Nutrition University of California, Davis http://cetulare.ucanr.edu/files/32432.pdf

Jane V. Higdon, Balz Frei, "Coffee and Health: A review of Recent Human Research" Critical Reviews in Food Science and Nutrition (2006) Vol. 46, Issue. 2, p. 101-123 DOI: 10.1080/10408390500400009

Rachel Johnson, Susan Bryant, Alyson L. Huntley, "Green tea and green tea catechin extracts: An overview of the clinical evidence" Maturitas, Vol. 73, Issue 4, p. 280-287

Tannis M Jurgens, Anne Marie Whelan, Lara Killian, Steve Doucette, Sara Kirk, Elizabeth Foy, "Green tea for weight loss and weight maintenance in overweight or obese adults." Cochrane Database of Systematic Reviews (12 December 2012), Issue 12, Art. No.: CD008650.

DOI: 10.1002/14651858.CD008650.pub2.

Shinichi Kuriyama, Taichi Shimazu, Kaori Ohmori, Nobutaka Kikuchi, Naoki Nakaya, Yoshikazu Nishino, Yoshitaka Tsubono, Ichiro Tsuji, "Green Tea Consumption and Mortality Due to Cardiovascular Disease, Cancer, and All Causes in Japan" (13 September 2006) JAMA. Vol 296, No.10, p.1255-1265. doi:10.1001/jama.296.10.1255

James D. Lane, Christina E. Barkauskas, Richard S. Surwit, Mark N. Feinglos, "Caffeine Impairs Glucose Metabolism in Type 2 Diabetes" Diabetes Care (27 August 2004) Vol. 8, p. 2047-2048 DOI: 10.2337/diacare.27.8.2047

Mayo Clinic "Caffeine: How much is too much?" (14 April 2014) http://www.mayoclinic.org/healthy-lifestyle/nutrition-and-healthy-eating/in-depth/caffeine/art-20045678

Filommenia Morisco, Vincenzo Lembo, Giovanna Mazzone, Silvia Camera, Nicola Caporaso, "Coffee and Liver Health" Journal of Clinical Gastroenterology (November/December 2014) Vol. 48, p. S87-S90. doi: 10.1097/MCG.0000000000000240

Wine/Alcoholic Beverages

Centers for Disease Control and Prevention, "Alcohol and Public Health – Frequently Asked Questions" (18 October 2016) https://www.cdc.gov/alcohol/faqs.htm

Gupta, A., Ellis, M.E., Oduse, K.A "The roles of phytochemicals in red wine as a protective agent against alcohol damage" International Food Research Journal (January 2013) Vol. 20, Issue 3, p. 1191-1197

What About Artificial Sweeteners?

Magalie Lenoir, Fuschia Serre, Lauriane Cantin, Serge H. Ahmed, "Intense Sweetness Surpasses Cocaine Reward" PLoS ONE. (2007) Vol. 2, No. 8, P. e698. doi: 10.1371/journal.pone.0000698.

Jennifer A. Nettleton, Pamela L. Lutsey, Youfa Wang, João A. Lima, Erin D. Michos, David R. Jacobs, "Diet Soda Intake and Risk of Incident Metabolic Syndrome and Type 2 Diabetes in the Multi-Ethnic Study of Atherosclerosis (MESA)" Diabetes Care (April 2009) Vol. 32, No. 4 p. 688-694. doi: 10.2337/dc08-1799

M. Yanina Pepino, Courtney D. Tiemann, Bruce W. Patterson, Burton M. Wice, Samuel Klein, "Sucralose Affects Glycemic and Hormonal Responses to an Oral Glucose Load" Diabetes Care (Sep 2013) Vol. 36, No. 9, p. 2530-2535. DOI: 10.2337/dc12-2221

Tim Spector, "Most of what we eat is 'processed' food. Here's why we should be worried" Spectator Health (4 July 2016) https://health.spectator.co.uk/most-of-what-we-eat-is-processed-food-heres-why-we-should-be-worried/

US Food and Drug administration, "Import Alert 45-06" (13 June 2016) http://www.accessdata.fda.gov/cms_ia/importalert_119.html

Tran's Fats and Refined Vegetable Oils

Saffron Alexander, "The oil guide: which to use for frying, drizzling and roasting" The Telegraph (10 NOVEMBER 2015) http://www.telegraph.co.uk/food-and-drink/healthy-eating/everything-you-know-about-cooking-with-oil-is-wrong/

Christinawaty, Sophi Damayanti, "Simultaneous Determination Method of BUTYLHYDROXYANISOLE, BUTYL HYDROXY TOLUENE, PROPYL GALLATE, ad TERTIARY BUTYL HYDROQUINONE in Margarine Using High Performance Liquid Chromatography" Asian Journal of Pharmaceutical and Clinical Research, (2015) Vol. 8, Issue 4, p. 209-211

Hyman, MD, Eat Fat, Get Thin (Little, Brown and Company Hachette Book Group, 2016) p. 17

Kamsiah Jaarin, Mohd Rais Mustafa, Xin-Fang Leong, "The effects of heated vegetable oils on blood pressure in rats. "Clinics. (2011) Vol. 66, No.12, p. 2125-2132. doi:10.1590/S1807-59322011001200020.

Robert Mendick, "Cooking with vegetable oils releases toxic cancer-causing chemicals, say experts" The Telegraph (07 Nov 2015) http://www.telegraph.co.uk/news/health/news/11981884/Cooking-with-vegetable-oils-releases-toxic-cancer-causing-chemicals-say-experts.html

Sunil Ratnayake, Paul Lewandowski, "Rapid bioassay-guided screening of toxic substances in vegetable oils that shorten the life of SHRSP rats" Lipids in Health and Disease (2010) Vol. 9, No.13, doi:10.1186/1476-511X-9-13.

Simopoulos, "The Importance of the Omega-6/Omega-3 Fatty Acid Ratio" Experimental Biology and Medicine (1 June 2008)

Soy Products

Breast Cancer Fund, "Phytoestrogens (Plant Estrogens)" (2016) http://www.breastcancerfund.org/clear-science/radiation-chemicals-and-breast-cancer/phytoestrogens.html

Heather B. Patisaul, Wendy Jefferson, "The pros and cons of phytoestrogens" Frontiers in Neuroendocrinology (October 2010) Vol. 31, No. 4, p.400-419. doi: 10.1016/j.yfrne.2010.03.003.

How You'll be Eating, and How Often. An Introduction to Mindful Eating.

Ingrid Elizabeth Lofgren, PhD, MPH, RD, "Mindful Eating" American Journal of Lifestyle Medicine (9 February 2015) American Journal of Lifestyle Medicine Vol 9, Issue 3, pp. 212-216

Mullin, The Gut Balance Revolution (Rodale Inc. 2014) p. 2-3

Eric Robinson, Paul Aveyard, Amanda Daley, Kate Jolly, Amanda Lewis, Deborah Lycett, Suzanne Higgs, "Eating attentively: a systematic review and meta-analysis of the effect of food intake memory and awareness on eating" The American Journal of Clinical Nutrition (April 2013) Vol. 97, No. 4, p. 728-742

Nina Van Dyke, Eric J Drinkwater, "Review Article Relationships between intuitive eating and health indicators: literature review" Public Health Nutrition, (August 2014) Vol. 17, No. 8, p. 1757-1766. doi: 10.1017/S1368980013002139.

For Pre-Diabetics and Those with Type 2 Diabetes

American Diabetes Association "Checking Your Blood Glucose"(4 August 2016) http://www.diabetes.org/living-with-diabetes/treatment-and-care/blood-glucose-control/checking-your-blood-glucose.html?referrer=https://www.google.com/

Mayo Clinic "Blood sugar testing: Why, when and how" (20 December 2014) http://www.mayoclinic.org/diseases-conditions/diabetes/in-depth/blood-sugar/art-20046628

Mayo Clinic "Type 2 diabetes" (13 January 2016) http://www.mayoclinic.org/diseases-conditions/type-2-diabetes/diagnosis-treatment/diagnosis/dxc-20169894

NIH National Institute of Diabetes and Digestive and Kidney Diseases "Diagnosis of Diabetes and Prediabetes" (June 2014) https://sp-web.niddk.nih.gov/health-information/health-topics/Diabetes/diagnosis-diabetes-prediabetes/Pages/index.aspx

Vitamins, Minerals, and Supplements

Eun Hee Koh, Woo Je Lee, Sang Ah Lee, Eun Hee Kim, Eun Hee Cho, Eunheui Jeong, Dong Woo Kim, Min-Seon Kim, Joong-Yeol Park, Keun-Gyu Park, Hyo-Jung Lee, In-Kyu Lee, Soo Lim, Hak Chul Jang, Ki Hoon Lee, Ki-Up Lee, "Effects of Alpha-Lipoic Acid on Body Weight in Obese Subjects" The American Journal of Medicine, Vol. 124, Issue 1, p. 85. e1-85. e8

Office of Disease Prevention and Health Promotion, "Scientific Report of the 2015 Dietary Guidelines Advisory Committee- Part D. Chapter 1: Food and Nutrient Intakes, and Health: Current Status and Trends" (2016) https://health.gov/dietaryguidelines/2015-scientific-report/PDFs/06-Part-D-Chapter-1.pdf

Gaia Pocobelli, Ulrike Peters, Alan R. Kristal, Emily White, "Use of Supplements of Multivitamins, Vitamin C, and Vitamin E in Relation to Mortality." American Journal of Epidemiology (2009) Vol. 170, No.4, p. 472-483. doi: 10.1093/aje/kwp167

Elizabeth Ward, "Addressing nutritional gaps with multivitamin and mineral supplements" Nutrition Journal (2014) Vol. 13, No. 72, doi: 10.1186/1475-2891-13-72

Qun Xu, Christine G Parks, Lisa A DeRoo, Richard M Cawthon, Dale P Sandler, and Honglei Chen, "Multivitamin use and telomere length in women" The American Journal of Clinical Nutrition (June 2009) Vol. 89, No. 6, p. 1857-1863

Alpha-Lipoic Acid

Jane Higdon, Victoria J. Drake, "Lipoic Acid" Oregon State University – Linus Pauling Institute Micronutrient Information Center (January 2012) http://lpi.oregonstate.edu/mic/dietary-factors/lipoic-acid

University of Maryland - Medical Center, "Alpha-lipoic acid" (26 June 2014) http://umm.edu/health/medical/altmed/supplement/alphalipoic-acid

WebMD, "Alpha Lipoic Acid (ALA)" (2016) http://www.webmd.com/diet/alpha-lipoic-acid-ala#1

Ashwagandha (Withania Somnifera)

eMedicineHealth, "Ashwagandha" (2016) p. 1-3 http://www.emedicinehealth.com/ashwagandha/vitamins-supplements.htm

Memorial Sloan Kettering Cancer Center, "Ashwagandha" (29 December 2015) https://www.mskcc.org/cancer-care/integrative-medicine/herbs/ashwagandha

Jaspal Singh Sandhu, Biren Shah, Shweta Shenoy, Suresh Chauhan, G. S. Lavekar, M. M. Padhi, "Effects of Withania somnifera (Ashwagandha) and Terminalia arjuna (Arjuna) on physical performance and cardiorespiratory endurance in healthy young adults" International Journal of Ayurveda Research (September 2010) Vol.1, Issue 3, p. 144-149. doi:10.4103/0974-7788.72485.

Narendra Singh, Mohit Bhalla, Prashanti de Jager, Marilena Gilca, "An Overview on Ashwagandha: A Rasayana (Rejuvenator) of Ayurveda" African Journal of Traditional, Complementary, and Alternative Medicines. (2011) Vol. 8, (5 Suppl.) p. 208-213. doi:10.4314/ajtcam.v8i5S.9.

Vitamin B Complex

MDhealth.Com, "Side Effects of Vitamin B Complex" (2 September 2016) http://www.md-health.com/Vitamin-B-Complex-Side-Effects.html

Med-Health.net, "Vitamin B Complex Benefits" (2 September 2016) http://www.med-health.net/B-Complex-Benefits.html

Medicine Net.com, "Vitamin b complex - oral, Nephro-vite, Nephrocaps, Triph" (August 2013) http://www.medicinenet.com/vitamin_b_complex-oral/article.htm

National Institutes of Health – Office of Dietary Supplements, "Vitamin B12 Dietary Supplement Fact Sheet" (11 February 2016) https://ods.od.nih.gov/factsheets/VitaminB12-HealthProfessional/university

Vitamin B12

Jane Higdon, Victoria J. Drake, Barbara Delage, "Vitamin B12" Oregon State University – Linus Pauling Institute Micronutrient Information Center (4 June 2016) http://lpi.oregonstate.edu/mic/vitamins/vitamin-B12

Mayo Clinic, "Drugs and Supplements Vitamin B12" (1 November 2013) http://www.mayoclinic.org/drugs-supplements/vitamin-b12/background/hrb-20060243

Patrick J. Skerrett, "Vitamin B12 deficiency can be sneaky, harmful" Harvard Health Blog (18 October 2016) http://www.health.harvard.edu/blog/vitamin-b12-deficiency-can-be-sneaky-harmful-201301105780

University of Maryland - Medical Center, "Vitamin B12 (Cobalamin)" (19 October 2015) http://umm.edu/health/medical/altmed/supplement/vitamin-b12-cobalamin

WebMD, "Find a Vitamin or Supplement – Vitamin B12" (2009) http://www.webmd.com/vitamins-supplements/ingredientmono-926-vitamin%20b12.aspx?activeingredientid=926

WebMD, "Vitamin B12 Deficiency" (23 July 2015) http://www.webmd.com/food-recipes/guide/vitamin-b12-deficiency-symptoms-causes#1

Vitamin D & Calcium

Heike A Bischoff-Ferrari, Bess Dawson-Hughes, John A Baron, Peter Burckhardt, Ruifeng Li, Donna Spiegelman, Bonny Specker, John E Orav, John B Wong, Hannes B Staehelin, Eilis O'Reilly, Douglas P Kiel, and Walter C Willett, "Calcium intake and hip fracture risk in men and women: a meta-analysis of prospective cohort studies and randomized controlled trials" The American Journal of Clinical Nutrition (December 2007) Vol. 86, No. 6, p. 1780-1790

Kevin D Cashman, Kirsten G Dowling, Zuzana Škrabáková, Marcela

Gonzalez-Gross, Jara Valtueña, Stefaan De Henauw, Luis Moreno, Camilla T Damsgaard, Kim F Michaelsen, Christian Mølgaard, Rolf Jorde, Guri Grimnes, George Moschonis, Christina Mavrogianni, Yannis Manios, Michael Thamm, Gert BM Mensink, Martina Rabenberg, Markus A Busch, Lorna Cox, Sarah Meadows, Gail Goldberg, Ann Prentice, Jacqueline M Dekker, Giel Nijpels, Stefan Pilz, Karin M Swart, Natasja M van Schoor, Paul Lips, Gudny Eiriksdottir, Vilmundur Gudnason, Mary Frances Cotch, Seppo Koskinen, Christel Lamberg-Allardt, Ramon A Durazo-Arvizu, Christopher T Sempos, and Mairead Kiely, "Vitamin D deficiency in Europe: pandemic?" The American Journal of Clinical Nutrition (2016) doi: 10.3945/ajcn.115.120873

Kimberly Y.Z. Forrest, Wendy L. Stuhldreher, "Prevalence and correlates of vitamin D deficiency in US adults" Nutrition Research, Vol. 31, Issue 1, p. 48-54

Harvard Health Publications - Harvard Medical School, "Vitamin D and your health: Breaking old rules, raising new hopes" (June 2009) http://www.health.harvard.edu/mens-health/vitamin-d-and-your-health

Harvard T.H. Chan School of Public Health, "The Nutrition Source - Vitamin D and Health" (2016) https://www.hsph.harvard.edu/nutritionsource/vitamin-d/

Michael F Holick, Tai C Chen, "Vitamin D deficiency: a worldwide problem with health consequences" The American Journal of Clinical Nutrition (April 2008) Vol. 87, No. 4, p. 1080s-1086s

University of Maryland - Medical Center, "Vitamin D – Overview" (2016) http://umm.edu/health/medical/altmed/supplement/vitamin-d

WebMD "Vitamin D: Uses, Side Effects, Interactions" (2016) http://www.webmd.com/vitamins-supplements/ingredientmono-929-vitamin%20d.aspx?activeingredientid=929

Rekha Mankad, "Calcium supplements: A risk factor for heart attack? - Mayo Clinic" Mayo Clinic (11 February 2016) http://www.

mayoclinic.org/diseases-conditions/heart-attack/expert-answers/calcium-supplements/faq-20058352

Magnesium

Cedars Sinai Medical Center, "Magnesium Rich Foods" (2016) https://www.cedars-sinai.edu/Patients/Programs-and-Services/Documents/CP0403MagnesiumRichFoods.pdf

Rebecca Costello, Taylor C Wallace, Andrea Rosanoff, "Nutrient Information: Magnesium" Advances in Nutrition p://www.encyclopedia.com/medicine/encyclopedias-almanacs-transcripts-and-maps/magnesium

Paul Hrkal, "Understanding Different types of Magnesium" Advanced Orthomolecular Research (9 September 2013) http://www.aor.ca/en/blog-details/understanding-different-types-of-magnesium

National Institutes of Health – Office of Dietary Supplements, "Magnesium Fact Sheet for Health Professionals" (2016) https://ods.od.nih.gov/factsheets/Magnesium-HealthProfessional/

University of Maryland - Medical Center, "Magnesium – Overview" (2016) http://umm.edu/health/medical/altmed/supplement/magnesium

WebMD "Magnesium" (2016) http://www.webmd.com/diet/supplement-guide-magnesium#1

Probiotics

Berkeley Wellness - University of California, "Probiotics Pros and Cons" (3 March 2014) http://www.berkeleywellness.com/supplements/other-supplements/article/probiotics-pros-and-cons

Thalis Ferreira dos Santos, Tauá Alves Melo, Milena Evangelista Almeida, Rachel Passos Rezende, Carla Cristina Romano, "Immunomodulatory Effects of Lactobacillus plantarum Lp62 on Intestinal Epithelial and Mononuclear Cells," BioMed Research International, (2016) Vol. 2016,

Article ID 8404156, 8 pages, doi:10.1155/2016/8404156

Karin Hove, Charlotte Brøns, Kristine Faerch, Søren Søgaard Lund, Peter Rossing, Allan Vaag, "Effects of 12 weeks treatment with fermented milk on blood pressure, glucose metabolism and markers of cardiovascular risk in patients with type 2 diabetes: a randomized double-blind placebo-controlled study." European Journal of Endocrinology, (9 October 2014) Vol. 172, p. 11-20, doi: 10.1530/EJE-14-0554

Valerio Mezzasalma, Enrico Manfrini, Emanuele Ferri, et al., "A Randomized, Double-Blind, Placebo-Controlled Trial: The Efficacy of Multispecies Probiotic Supplementation in Alleviating Symptoms of Irritable Bowel Syndrome Associated with Constipation," BioMed Research International, (2016) Vol. 2016, Article ID 4740907, 10 pages. doi:10.1155/2016/4740907

Mary Ellen Sanders, "Probiotics: Definition, Sources, Selection, and Uses." Clinical Infectious Diseases (2008) Vol. 46, Supplement 2, p. S58-S61. doi: 10.1086/523341

Marie-Agnès Travers, Isabelle Florent, Linda Kohl, Philippe Grellier, "Probiotics for the Control of Parasites: An Overview," Journal of Parasitology Research, (2011) Vol. 2011, Article ID 610769, 11 pages. doi:10.1155/2011/610769

University of Wisconsin Integrative Medicine, "Probiotics and Prebiotics: Frequently Asked Questions" (2016) http://www.fammed.wisc.edu/files/webfm-uploads/documents/outreach/im/handout_probiotics_patient.pdf

Sarah H. Yi, John A. Jernigan, L. Clifford McDonald, "Prevalence of probiotic use among inpatients: A descriptive study of 145 U.S. hospitals" American Journal of Infection Control (1 May 2016) Vol. 44, Issue 5, p. 548–553

Rhodiola Rosea

Richard P. Brown, M.D., Patricia L. Gerbarg, M.D., Barbara Graham, The Rhodiola Revolution (Rodale 2004)

Tulsi/Holy Basil

Melissa Eisler, "What is Holy Basil?" The Chopra Center (2016) http://www.chopra.com/articles/what-is-holy-basil#sm.0000a0fg6d6qve k2qui1z1cj7im1l

Michigan Medicine University of Michigan, "Holy Basil" (2016) http://www.uofmhealth.org/health-library/hn-4597000

WebMD, "Find a Vitamin or Supplement – Holy Basil"(2016) http://www.webmd.com/vitamins-supplements/ingredientmono-1101-holy%20basil.aspx?activeingredientid=1101

Life Style Strategies

Lise Alschuler, "Optimal Longevity Hinges on Telomeres" Natural Medicine Journal (June 2013) Vol. 5, Issue 6, (ISSN 2157-6769) http://www.naturalmedicinejournal.com/journal/2013-06/optimal-longevity-hinges-telomeres

Genetic Science Learning Center. "Are Telomeres the Key to Aging and Cancer." Learn. Genetics. (1 March 2016) http://learn.genetics.utah.edu/content/basics/telomeres/.

Eli Puterman, Jue Lin, Jeffrey Krauss, Elizabeth H. Blackburn, Elissa S. Epel, "Determinants of telomere attrition over 1 year in healthy older women: stress and health behaviors matter" Molecular psychiatry. (April 2015) Vol. 20, No. 4, p. 529-535. doi:10.1038/mp.2014.70.

Masood A. Shammas, "Telomeres, lifestyle, cancer, and aging" Current Opinion in Clinical Nutrition and Metabolic Care. (January 2011) Vol. 14, No. 1 p. 28-34. doi:10.1097/MCO.0b013e32834121b1.

Getting Enough Sleep, the More You Know...

American Psychological Association, "Getting a good night's sleep" (2016) http://www.apa.org/helpcenter/sleep-disorders.aspx

Harvard Medical School Division of Sleep Medicine, "Twelve Simple Tips to Improve Your Sleep" (18 December 2007) http://healthysleep.med.harvard.edu/healthy/getting/overcoming/tips

Marie-Pierre St-Onge, Amy Roberts, Ari Shechter, Arindam Roy Choudhury, "Fiber and saturated fat are associated with sleep arousals and slow wave sleep." Journal of Clinical Sleep Medicine (2016) Vol.12, No. 1, p.19-24

National Institute on Aging, "Age Page - A Good Night's Sleep" (May 2016) https://www.nia.nih.gov/health/publication/good-nights-sleep

Sleep Apnea

Mayo Clinic, "Diseases and Conditions – Sleep apnea" (25 August 2015) http://www.mayoclinic.org/diseases-conditions/sleep-apnea/basics/definition/con-20020286

Restless Leg Syndrome (RLS)

NIH National Institute of Neurological Disorders and Stroke, "Restless Legs Syndrome Fact Sheet"(September 2010) NIH Publication No. 10-4847 https://www.ninds.nih.gov/Disorders/Patient-Caregiver-Education/Fact-Sheets/Restless-Legs-Syndrome-Fact-Sheet

National Sleep Foundation, "Restless Legs Syndrome (RLS) Symptoms" (2016) https://sleepfoundation.org/content/restless-legs-syndrome-rls-symptoms

Periodic Limb Disorder

National Institute on Aging, "Age Page - A Good Night's Sleep" (May 2016) https://www.nia.nih.gov/health/publication/good-nights-sleep

Taking a Load Off

Mayo Clinic Healthy lifestyle, "Chronic stress puts your health at risk" (21 April 2016) http://www.mayoclinic.org/healthy-lifestyle/stress-management/in-depth/stress/art-20046037

Exercise

Centers for Disease Control and Prevention, "Healthy Places – Physical Activity" (4 February 2016) https://www.cdc.gov/healthyplaces/healthtopics/physactivity.htm

Dan M. Sullivan, "Endorphins - Chemistry: Foundations and Applications" Encyclopedia.com. (2004) http://www.encyclopedia.com/science-and-technology/biochemistry/biochemistry/endorphins

Yoga

Timothy Burgin, "History of Yoga" Yoga Basics (2015) http://www.yogabasics.com/learn/history-of-yoga/

Sujit Chandratreya, "Yoga: An evidence-based therapy." Journal of Mid-Life Health. (2011) Vol. 2, No. 1, p. 3-4. doi:10.4103/0976-7800.83251.

Braden Kuo, Manoj Bhasin, Jolene Jacquart, Matthew A. Scult, Lauren Slipp, Eric Isaac Kagan Riklin, Veronique Lepoutre, Nicole Comosa, Beth-Ann Norton, Allison Dassatti, Jessica Rosenblum, Andrea H. Thurler, Brian C. Surjanhata, Nicole N. Hasheminejad, Leslee Kagan, Ellen Slawsby, Sowmya R. Rao, Eric A. Macklin, Gregory L. Fricchione, Herbert Benson, Towia A. Libermann, Joshua Korzenik, John W. Denninge, "Genomic and Clinical Effects Associated with a Relaxation Response Mind-Body Intervention in Patients with Irritable Bowel Syndrome and Inflammatory Bowel Disease" (30 April 2015) PLoS ONE Vol. 10, No. 4, e0123861. doi:10.1371/journal.pone.0123861

Reference, "How old is yoga?" (2017) https://www.reference.com/health/old-yoga-68a54696e23b84e1#

Catherine Woodyard, "Exploring the therapeutic effects of yoga and its ability to increase quality of life." International Journal of Yoga. (2011) Vol. 4, No. 2, p. 49-54. doi:10.4103/0973-6131.85485.

Meditation

Institute of Noetic Sciences, "Meditation Types" (2016) http://www.noetic.org/meditation-bibliography/meditation-types

Relaxation Yoga

Adam Brady, "10 Benefits of Restorative Yoga" The Chopra Center (2016) http://www.chopra.com/articles/10-benefits-of-restorative-yoga#sm.0000a0fg6d6qvek2qui1z1cj7im1l

DoYogaWithMe, "14 Different Yoga Styles and Their Benefits to Your Health" (2017) https://www.doyogawithme.com/types-of-yoga

Do That Thing You Love Doing

Dyer, W., Wayne Dyer: 10 principles / The power of intention, Laurent Puechguirbal; You Tube (April 12, 2012) https://youtu.be/xip3YjSTZlU

Don't Worry Needlessly

Dyer, W., Wayne Dyer Your Erroneous Zones Full Audiobook, Gift Essentials; You Tube (September 5, 2015) https://youtu.be/VaM5L-z5Kgw?list=PLF8pwIT0dxjtNStoY2LpuCDiBq1gsEFwy

Focusing on the Positive

Robert A. Emmons, Michael E. McCullough, "Counting Blessings Versus Burdens: An Experimental Investigation of Gratitude and

Subjective Well-Being in Daily Life" Journal of Personality and Social Psychology, (Feb 2003) Vol 84, No. 2, p. 377-389

Robert A. Emmons, Robin Stern, "Gratitude as a Psychotherapeutic Intervention" Journal of Clinical Psychology (August 2013) Vol.69, Issue 8, p. 846–855

Paul J. Mills, Laura Redwine, Kathleen Wilson, Meredith A. Pung, Kelly Chinh, Barry H. Greenberg, Ottar Lunde, Alan Maisel, Ajit Raisinghani, Alex Wood, Deepak Chopra, "The Role of Gratitude in Spiritual Well-being in Asymptomatic Heart Failure Patients" Spirituality in clinical practice (2015) Vol. 2, No. 1, p.5-17. doi:10.1037/scp0000050.

Alex M. Wood, Stephen Joseph, John Maltby, "Gratitude predicts psychological well-being above the Big Five facets" Personality and Individual Differences (2009) Vol. 46, No. 4, p. 443-447.

Take Five

North Shore University Health System, "Ten Natural Ways to Manage Your Stress Levels" (02 November 2016) http://www.northshore.org/healthy-you/ten-natural-ways-to-manage-stress/

Friends, Family, and Community

Sheldon Cohen, Denise Janicki-Deverts, Ronald B. Turner, William J. Doyle, "Does Hugging Provide Stress-Buffering Social Support? A Study of Susceptibility to Upper Respiratory Infection and Illness" (19 December 2014) Psychological Science Vol 26, Issue 2, p. 135-147

Julianne Holt-Lunstad, Wendy A. Birmingham, Kathleen C. Light, "Influence of a "warm touch" support enhancement intervention among married couples on ambulatory blood pressure, oxytocin, alpha amylase, and cortisol." Psychosomatic Medicine (November 2008) Vol. 70, No.9, p. 976-985 doi: 10.1097/PSY.0b013e318187aef7

NIH News in Health, "The Power of Love - Hugs and Cuddles Have

Long-Term Effects" (February 2007) https://newsinhealth.nih.gov/2007/february/docs/01features_01.htm

GLOSSARY OF TERMS

Allergens: a substance that induces allergy

Alopecia: partial or complete loss of hair

Alzheimer's: a degenerative brain disease of unknown cause that is the most common form of dementia, that usually starts in late middle age or in old age, that results in progressive memory loss, impaired thinking, disorientation, and changes in personality and mood, and that is marked histologically by the degeneration of brain neurons especially in the cerebral cortex and by the presence of neurofibrillary tangles and plaques containing beta-amyloid —abbreviation AD

Angina: a heart disease that causes brief periods of intense chest pain

Antioxidants: any of various substances (as beta-carotene, vitamin C, and alpha-tocopherol) that inhibit oxidation or reactions promoted by oxygen and peroxides and that include many held to protect the living body from the deleterious effects of free radicals

Arteriosclerosis: a chronic disease characterized by abnormal thickening and hardening of the arterial walls with resulting loss of elasticity

Arthritis: inflammation of joints due to infectious, metabolic, or constitutional causes

Atrophy: decrease in size or wasting away of a body part or tissue; also: arrested development or loss of a part or organ incidental to the normal development or life of an animal or plant

Autism Spectrum Disorder: any of a group of developmental disorders (such as autism and Asperger's syndrome) marked by impairments in the ability to communicate and interact socially and by the presence of repetitive behaviors or restricted interests

Autoimmune disease: a disease in which the body produces antibodies that attack its own tissues, leading to the deterioration and in some cases to the destruction of such tissue

Biological: of or relating to biology or to life and living processes

Cancer: a malignant tumor of potentially unlimited growth that expands locally by invasion and systemically by metastasis

Carcinogenesis: the production of cancer

Cardiac arrest: abrupt temporary or permanent cessation of the heartbeat (as from ventricular fibrillation or asystole)—called also sudden cardiac arrest

Chromosome: any of the rod-shaped or threadlike DNA-containing structures of cellular organisms that are located in the nucleus of eukaryotes, are usually ring-shaped in prokaryotes (as bacteria), and contain all or most of the genes of the organism; also: the genetic material of a virus

Chronic disease: a disease that persists for a long time. A chronic disease is one lasting 3 months or more, by the definition of the U.S. National Center for Health Statistics

Chronic illness: an illness that lasts 3 months or more

Chronic Inflammation: inflammation that may have a rapid or slow onset but is characterized primarily by its persistence and lack of clear resolution; it occurs when the tissues are unable to overcome the effects of the injuring agent

Chronic Fatigue Syndrome: a debilitating and complex disorder characterized by profound fatigue that is not improved by bed rest and that may be worsened by physical or mental activity.

Cirrhosis of the Liver: widespread disruption of normal liver structure by fibrosis and the formation of regenerative nodules that is caused by any of various chronic progressive conditions affecting the liver (as long-term alcohol abuse or hepatitis)

Commensal microflora: an organism participating in a symbiotic relationship in which one species derives some benefit while the other is unaffected

Congestive heart failure: heart failure in which the heart is unable to maintain adequate circulation of blood in the tissues of the body or to pump out the venous blood returned to it by the venous circulation

Cortisol: a glucocorticoid $C_{21}H_{30}O_5$ produced by the adrenal cortex upon stimulation by ACTH that mediates various metabolic processes (as gluconeogenesis), has anti-inflammatory and immunosuppressive properties, and whose levels in the blood may become elevated in response to physical or psychological stress

Cytokines: any of a class of immunoregulatory proteins (as interleukin or interferon) that are secreted by cells especially of the immune system

Diabetes Mellitus Type 2: diabetes mellitus of a common form that develops especially in adults and most often in obese individuals and that is characterized by hyperglycemia resulting from impaired insulin utilization coupled with the body's inability to compensate with increased insulin production—called also adult-onset diabetes, late-onset diabetes, maturity-onset diabetes, non-insulin-dependent diabetes, non-insulin-dependent diabetes mellitus, type 2 diabetes mellitus

Diuretic: an agent that increases the excretion of urine

Dysbiosis: a microbial imbalance or maladaptation on or inside the body

Emphysema: a condition characterized by air-filled expansions in interstitial or subcutaneous tissues; specifically: a condition of the lung that is marked by distension and eventual rupture of the alveoli with progressive loss of pulmonary elasticity, that is accompanied by shortness of breath with or without cough, and that may lead to impairment of heart action

Endocrinologist: a branch of medicine concerned with the structure, function, and disorders of the endocrine glands

Endothelium: an epithelium of mesoblastic origin composed of a single layer of thin flattened cells that lines internal body cavities

Enteric microflora: bacteria which reside in the intestines

Endorphins: any of a group of endogenous peptides (as enkephalin and dynorphin) found especially in the brain that bind chiefly to opiate receptors and produce some of the same pharmacological effects (as pain relief) as those of opiates

Endotoxin: a toxin of internal origin; specifically: a poisonous substance present in bacteria (as the causative agent of typhoid fever) but separable from the cell body only on its disintegration

Essential fatty acids: unsaturated fatty acids that are essential to human health, but cannot be manufactured in the body

Estrogen: any of various natural steroids (as estradiol) that are formed from androgen precursors, that are secreted chiefly by the ovaries, placenta, adipose tissue, and testes, and that stimulate the development of female secondary sex characteristics and promote the growth and maintenance of the female reproductive system

Free radicals: an especially reactive atom or group of atoms that has one or more unpaired electrons; especially: one that is produced in the body by natural biological processes or introduced from outside (as in tobacco smoke, toxins, or pollutants) and that can damage cells, proteins, and DNA by altering their chemical structure

Gastroenterology: a branch of medicine concerned with the structure, functions, diseases, and pathology of the stomach and intestines

Gastroesophageal Reflux Disease: a highly variable chronic condition that is characterized by periodic episodes of gastroesophageal reflux usually accompanied by heartburn and that may result in histopathologic changes in the esophagus—called also GERD

GERD: gastroesophageal reflux disease

Gene: a specific sequence of nucleotides in DNA or RNA that is located usually on a chromosome and that is the functional unit of inheritance controlling the transmission and expression of one or more traits by specifying the structure of a particular polypeptide and especially a protein or controlling the function of other genetic material—called also determinant, determiner, factor

Ghrelin: a 28-amino-acid peptide hormone that is secreted primarily by stomach cells with lesser amounts secreted by other cells (as of the pancreas) and acts to stimulate appetite and the secretion of growth hormone

Glycemia: the presence of glucose in the blood

Gout: a metabolic disease marked by a painful inflammation of the joints, deposits of urates in and around the joints, and usually an excessive amount of uric acid in the blood

Heart Disease: an abnormal organic condition of the heart or of the heart and circulation

Hormone: a product of living cells that circulates in body fluids (as blood) or sap and produces a specific often stimulatory effect on the activity of cells usually a distance from its point of synthesis

Hypertension: abnormally high blood pressure and especially arterial blood pressure

Hyperinsulinemia: the presence of excess insulin in the blood

Inflammatory Bowel Disease: either of two inflammatory diseases of the bowel:

1. Crohn's disease
2. ulcerative colitis

Insulin: a protein pancreatic hormone secreted by the beta cells of the islets of Langerhans that is essential especially for the metabolism of carbohydrates and the regulation of glucose levels in the blood and that when insufficiently produced results in diabetes mellitus

Insulin-degrading enzyme: an enzyme secreted by cells to mitigate insulin in the blood.

Insulin resistance: reduced sensitivity to insulin by the body's insulin-dependent processes (as glucose uptake and lipolysis) that is typical of type 2 diabetes but often occurs in the absence of diabetes

Leptin: a peptide hormone that is produced by fat cells and plays a role in body weight regulation by acting on the hypothalamus to suppress appetite and burn fat stored in adipose tissue

Lipopolysaccharide: also known as lipoglycans and endotoxins, are large molecules consisting of a lipid and a polysaccharide; they are found in the outer membrane of Gram-negative bacteria, and elicit strong immune responses in animals

Macronutrient: a substance (as a protein, carbohydrate, or fat) required in relatively large quantities for growth, energy, and health

Malnutrition: deficiencies, excesses, or imbalances in a person's intake of energy and/or nutrients

Metabolic rate: metabolism per unit time especially as estimated by food consumption, energy released as heat, or oxygen used in metabolic processes

Metabolic syndrome: a syndrome marked by the presence of usually three or more of a group of factors (as high blood pressure, abdominal obesity, high triglyceride levels, low HDL levels, and high fasting levels of blood sugar) that are linked to an increased risk of cardiovascular disease and type 2 diabetes—called also insulin resistance syndrome, syndrome X Metabolism

Microbiome: the trillions of microorganisms that live in and on our bodies.

Multigenic: controlled by or involving more than one gene

Neuroendocrinology: a branch of science dealing with neurosecretion and the physiological interaction between the central nervous system and the endocrine system

Nitroglycerin: a heavy oily explosive poisonous liquid $C_3H_5N_3O_9$ used chiefly in making dynamites and in medicine as a vasodilator (as in angina pectoris)—called also *trinitrin, trinitroglycerin*

Non-alcoholic fatty liver disease: a buildup of fat in the liver

Non-alcoholic steatohepatitis: an accumulation of excess fat, inflammation, damage, and scarring, in the liver of people who drink little or no alcohol

Obesity: a condition that is characterized by excessive accumulation and storage of fat in the body and that in an adult is typically indicated by a body mass index of 30 or greater

Pancreas: a large lobulated gland of vertebrates that secretes digestive enzymes and the hormones insulin and glucagon

Pathogenesis: the origination and development of a disease

Phyla: a genetically related group

Pneumonia: an acute disease that is marked by inflammation of lung tissue accompanied by infiltration of alveoli and often bronchioles with white blood cells (such as neutrophils) and fibrinous exudate, is characterized by fever, chills, cough, difficulty in breathing, fatigue, chest pain, and reduced lung expansion, and is typically caused by an infectious agent (such as a bacterium, virus, or fungus)

Prebiotic: a substance and especially a carbohydrate (such as inulin) that is nearly or wholly indigestible and that when consumed (as in food) promotes the growth of beneficial bacteria in the digestive tract

Pulmonary Hypertension: high blood pressure in the pulmonary arteries that can lead to severe shortness of breath and death

Refined carbohydrates: plant-based foods that have the whole grain extracted during processing

Resting metabolic rate: the minimum number of calories needed to support basic functions, including breathing and circulation

Restless leg syndrome: a disorder characterized by an unpleasant tickling or twitching sensation in the leg muscles when sitting or lying down, relieved only by moving the legs

Serotonin: a neurotransmitter that is involved in sleep, depression, memory, and other neurological processes

Sleep apnea: a temporary cessation of breathing during sleep

Symbiotic microflora: bacteria living in symbiosis with another organism or each other

Symbiosis: interaction between two different organisms living in close physical association, typically to the advantage of both

Telomere: the natural end of a eukaryotic chromosome composed of a usually repetitive DNA sequence and serving to stabilize the chromosome

Testosterone: a steroid hormone that stimulates development of male secondary sexual characteristics, produced mainly in the testes, but also in the ovaries and adrenal cortex

Thermodynamics: physics that deals with the mechanical action or relations of heat

Thyroid: a large bilobed endocrine gland of craniate vertebrates that arises as a median ventral outgrowth of the pharynx, lies in the anterior base of the neck or anterior ventral part of the thorax, produces especially the hormones thyroxine and triiodothyronine

Type 2 Diabetes: diabetes mellitus of a common form that develops especially in adults and most often in obese individuals and that is characterized by hyperglycemia resulting from impaired insulin utilization coupled with the body's inability to compensate with increased insulin production

Urea nitrogen: a waste product from the breakdown of protein in the body

RECIPE INDEX

613.25 BOM

Bomzer, Lee
Healthy body
 connection : unlocking

08/23/18

CPSIA information can be obtained
at www.ICGtesting.com
Printed in the USA
LVOW13s0327190218
566954LV00003B/3/P